Re/Imagining Depression

"As anxiety and depression become the bedrock of our everyday lives, we urgently need these essays, which investigate the limits of 'mental health' as a frame for addressing social and political violence. Drawing on rich resources of art and theory, these writers offer hope for a collective future—while taking despair seriously. A darkly utopian vision for our time."

—Heather Love, *Professor, English, University of Pennsylvania, USA. Author of* Feeling Backward: Loss and the Politics of Queer History (2007)

"Western medical discourse and the glut of pills it prescribes have long dominated our conceptions of depression. In this welcome collection, Hollenbach and McDonald have assembled a compelling arsenal of creativity against the 'war on worries.' Turning to arts and humanities—to literature, poetry, performance, and visual cultural—*Re/Imagining Depression* creates a new language for sadness that reengages it for hope and change."

—David L. Eng, *Professor, English, University of Pennsylvania, USA. Author of* The Feeling of Kinship: Queer Liberalism and the Racialization of Intimacy (2010) and co-author of Racial Melancholia, Racial Dissociation: On the Social and Psychic Lives of Asian Americans (2019)

"This compilation of writing on depression and art could not have come at a more perfect time. The book brings conversations about the practices of self (and collective) care alongside the practices of art making into a fulsome and rich collection where no one stands alone and we work to think these complex relationships through together. The book is a deep dive into feelings and their implications—creating a useful rumination on making/remaking and how to keep going—keep living."

—Allyson Mitchell, *Artist, Co-Director of the Feminist Art Gallery, and Associate Professor, Gender Studies, York University, Canada. Creator of* Killjoy's Kastle: A Lesbian Feminist Haunted House

"How can we disentangle our bad feelings from the biomedical frameworks within which they are now almost always treated and understood? This question, so timely and important, is at the centre of the essays collected in this ground-breaking new study of depression. Robin Alex McDonald and Julie Hollenbach bring together a series of papers that each interrogate intersections between depression and race, gender and sexuality. Collectively, they rethink negative feelings outside bio-medical discourses of pathologisation. *Re/Imagining Depression: Creative Approaches to 'Feeling Bad'* offers productive and creative new ways to think about and with bad feelings, and to recognise the extent to which these are embedded in the textures and structures of everyday life."

—Elizabeth Stephens, *Associate Professor, Humanities and Social Sciences, University of Queensland, Australia. Author of* Anatomy as Spectacle: Public Exhibitions of the Body from 1700 to the Present (2011), *and co-author of* A Critical Genealogy of Normality (2017)

"It's clear that capitalism makes us feel bad and then makes us feel bad about feeling bad. We thus need to challenge capitalism on both levels. We need alternatives to the biomedical models and ideological discourses that dominate the world, pathologizing and personalizing the problem of depression. We need, desperately need, an anthology like *Re/Imagining Depression*."

—Mikkel Krause Frantzen, *Postdoctoral Fellow, Copenhagen University, Denmark. Author of* Going Nowhere, Slow: The Aesthetics and Politics of Depression (2019)

"When I was doing research for Rock Steady, it became painfully clear that I'd need to go well out of my way to find information outside of the 'imperialist white supremacist capitalist cisnormative heteronormative patriarchy' (Laverne Cox). I wish I'd had a copy of *Re/Imagining Depression*, for the eye-opening points of view, introductions to fascinating contemporary and historical figures, and inspirational lists of cited research and literature."

—Ellen Forney, *Instructor at the Cornish College of the Arts, USA. Author and illustrator of* Marbles: Mania, Depression, Michelangelo, & Me (2012) and Rock Steady: Brilliant Advice From My Bipolar Life (2018)

"This wonderful book seeks to collate a body of writing that disrupts the established conceptualisation of 'depression,' using an array of discourses and metaphors to interrogate boundaries of understanding. Poetically and critically, it punches a hole in the wall of psychiatry and its epistemological border checks. Its rich array of writing reveals how psychiatry marks certain voices and ideas as incomprehensible and turns these away for not holding a passport of preferred thinking. It promotes imagination as a valid entry qualification to depression and its meanings—for people."

—Paul Crawford, *Professor and Director of the Centre for Social Futures at the Institute of Mental Health, The University of Nottingham, UK. Author of* Madness in Post-1945 British and American Fiction (2010) *and co-author of* Health Humanities (2015)

"This is a powerful and welcome contribution to the urgent project of widening our understanding and treatment of depression (more properly depressions). Through a mix of academic and creative essays, the contributors analyse depression as a profoundly political phenomenon."

—Clark Lawlor, *Professor, Humanities, Northumbria University, UK. Author of* From Melancholia to Prozac: a History of Depression (2012)

Julie Hollenbach · Robin Alex McDonald
Editors

Re/Imagining Depression

Creative Approaches to "Feeling Bad"

palgrave
macmillan

Editors
Julie Hollenbach
Art History and Contemporary Culture
NSCAD University
Halifax, NS, Canada

Robin Alex McDonald
Fine and Performing Arts
Nipissing University
North Bay, ON, Canada

ISBN 978-3-030-80553-1 ISBN 978-3-030-80554-8 (eBook)
https://doi.org/10.1007/978-3-030-80554-8

Cover illustration: Marcos Guinoza, Mind and Heart, 2020. Mixed digital collage and graphic design.

This Palgrave Macmillan imprint is published by the registered company Springer Nature Switzerland AG
The registered company address is: Gewerbestrasse 11, 6330 Cham, Switzerland

Acknowledgments

The editors would like to thank Camille Davies, Liam McLean, Jack Heeney, and everyone else at Palgrave Macmillan who believed in this project and helped to make it possible, as well as our intrepid indexer Nicole Marcoux.

Julie Hollenbach would like to thank NSCAD University and the Social Sciences and Humanities Research Council for their financial support in reprinting José Esteban Muñoz's "Feeling Brown, Feeling Down: Latina Affect, the Performativity of Race, and the Depressive Position," as well as providing funds toward the indexing of this volume.

Robin Alex McDonald would like to thank Nipissing University for their financial support in reprinting Nyasha Junior's "Don't We Hurt Like You? Examining the Lack of Portrayals of African American Women and Mental Health."

Finally, the editors would like to thank all of the contributors to *Re/Imagining Depression: Creative Approaches to "Feeling Bad,"* who have been patient and persevering throughout the process of assembling this book, which was destined to be published on crip time.

Contents

Notes on Contributors

Marie Allitt is a Humanities and Healthcare Fellow at the University of Oxford, and Postdoctoral Research Assistant for the Northern Network for Medical Humanities Research, at the University of Leeds, UK. She is an interdisciplinary researcher in medical/health/healthcare humanities and medical education. Marie completed her Ph.D. in English Literature at the University of York in 2018, focusing on experiences and representations of spaces and senses in the First World War medical caregiving narratives, with a monograph forthcoming. Marie's research focuses on medical life writing; practitioner health; trauma and mental health; early twentieth-century surgery; senses; and medical spaces, architectures, and environments.

Pansee Atta is an Egyptian-Canadian visual artist, curator, and researcher living and working on the unceded territory of the Algonquin Anishnaabe nation in Ottawa. Her work examines themes of representation, migration, archives, and political struggle. Her curatorial work includes UTOPIAS, a community-based performance art festival in Kingston, Ontario and Home/Making at the Canada Council Art Bank. Previous residencies have taken place at the Montréal Museum of Fine Arts, SparkBox Studio, and the Atelier of Alexandria. Exhibitions of her artwork have taken place at the Modern Fuel Artist-Run Centre, Galerie La Centrale Powerhouse, Z Art Space, the Art Gallery of Mississauga, and other contemporary Canadian arts spaces. Her SSHRC-funded doctoral research examines decolonial museum practices in the Middle East.

Hamish Ballantyne is a writer from Vancouver Island. He is a mental health worker and works seasonally as a mushroom picker. He recently finished translating *The Solitudes* by Luis de Góngora.

Jes Battis teaches medieval literature, creative writing, and queer things in the Department of English at the University of Regina. Recent publications include a book chapter on queer food studies (*Canadian Culinary Imaginations*, McGill-Queen's University Press) and an article on neurodiversity in popular culture (*Los Angeles Review of Books*). Their current monograph, *Thinking Queerly*, explores neurodiversity in medieval texts and is forthcoming from the Medieval Institute Press at the University of Western Michigan. Jes is also the author of the *Occult Special Investigator* series and *Parallel Parks* series, both with Ace/Penguin.

Feel Tank Chicago (Lauren Berlant; Romi N. Crawford; Mary Patten; Matthias Regan) is an art/activist group agitating and reconsidering political emotion since 2002. We explore intensities and events of political feeling. In performance, criticism, art, and activism, we focus on the political potential of "bad feelings" like hopelessness, apathy, anxiety, fear, numbness, despair, and ambivalence. Our sense of the political is on the streets and sidewalks, in the world, in the eruptive and the everyday... Writing, art-making, pedagogy, performance, and activism are all threads of our praxis. So is hope. http://www.feeltankchicago.net.

Ann Cvetkovich is the Director of Women's and Gender Studies, The Pauline Jewett Institute at Carleton University and formerly held the position of Ellen Clayton Garwood Centennial Professor of English and Professor of Women's and Gender Studies at the University of Texas at Austin. She is the author of *Mixed Feelings: Feminism, Mass Culture, and Victorian Sensationalism* (Rutgers, 1992); *An Archive of Feelings: Trauma, Sexuality, and Lesbian Public Cultures* (Duke, 2003); and *Depression: A Public Feeling* (Duke, 2012). She co-edited (with Ann Pellegrini) "Public Sentiments," a special issue of *The Scholar and Feminist Online*, and (with Janet Staiger and Ann Reynolds) *Political Emotions* (Routledge, 2010). She has been co-editor, with Annamarie Jagose, of *GLQ: A Journal of Lesbian and Gay Studies*. Her current writing projects focus on the current state of LGBTQ archives and the creative use of them by artists to create counterarchives and interventions in public history.

Francesca Ekwuyasi is a writer and multidisciplinary artist from Lagos, Nigeria. Her work explores themes of faith, family, queerness, consumption, loneliness, and belonging.

Her short documentary *Black + Belonging* screened at the Halifax Black Film Festival, Festival International du Film Black de Montréal, and Toronto Black Film Festival. You may find some of her writing in *Winter Tangerine Review, Brittle Paper, Transition Magazine, the Malahat Review, Visual Art News, Vol. 1 Brooklyn, GUTS magazine,* and elsehwere. Her story *Ọrun is Heaven* was longlisted for the 2019 Journey Prize and her debut novel *Butter Honey Pig Bread* (Arsenal Pulp Press, 2020) was longlisted for the Giller Prize.

Sima Godfrey is a specialist in nineteenth-century French literature and cultural history where she has published on all the usual suspects as well as some unusual ones. In addition to her current work on cultural memory, she has an ongoing interest in authors who were also art critics and theorists. Her most recent article in this vein appeared in *Brooklyn Rail,* Critics Page, "Hasards de la rime" (October 2019).

Julie Hollenbach is an Assistant Professor of Craft History and Material Culture at NSCAD University (Kjipuktuk/Halifax, NS). Her research is grounded in a queer, feminist, anti-racist, and decolonial methodologies, and considers cultural practices at the intersections of history and location, tradition and ritual, contact and connection, meaning and use. Hollenbach's writing has been published in popular press platforms such as *Canadian Art*, *Studio Magazine*, and *VANS*, as well as scholarly publications including *PUBLIC*, *Craft and Design*, and *Cahiers métiers d'art ::: Craft Journal*. Hollenbach has curated exhibitions at the Art Gallery of Nova Scotia, MSVU Art Gallery, Union Gallery, and the Anna Leonowens Gallery.

Alyson Hoy holds a Ph.D. in Curriculum and Instruction from the University of British Columbia. Working at the intersection of memoir writing and queer and feminist theories of feeling and embodiment, her writing explores themes of sex, queer identity, trauma, psychic life, anorexia, and self-harm. Her current project is a book manuscript of her doctoral dissertation. In this work, she draws on Eve Kosofsky Sedgwick's notion of the reparative, which seeks a different way of being and holding space in the world, as a means to intervene into theories of negativity that have become pervasive in queer theory, and to interrupt normative, medicalized accounts of illness and embodiment. Methodologically, she incorporates memoir and critical essay in ways that reference Sedgwick's innovative use of form and aim to open up new identifications and avenues for thinking about the experience of anorexia as an illness that is oriented to life and not only death. Her work refuses the western medical view of anorexia as a "pathology" triggered by forces that are mostly external to the subject and instead examines the intricacies of anorexic subjectivity, tracing the embodied and felt dimensions of anorexia and positing anorexia as a form of queer self-knowledge.

Nyasha Junior is a biblical scholar. She writes, teaches, speaks, and frequently tweets on religion, race, gender, and their intersections. She is the author of *An Introduction to Womanist Biblical Interpretation* (Westminster John Knox Press, 2015) and *Reimagining Hagar: Blackness and Bible* (Oxford University Press, 2019) and the co-author of *Black Samson: The Untold Story of an American Icon* (Oxford University Press, 2020).

Ken Lum is an artist who has participated in Documenta, the Venice Biennale, Sao Paolo Bienal, Shanghai Biennale, Istanbul Biennial, Gwangju Biennale, and Whitney Biennial.

He is Co-Founder and Founding Editor of *Yishu Journal of Contemporary Chinese Art*. He gave keynote addresses for the 2020 Markham Public Art Conference, 2010 World Museums Conference in Shanghai, the 2006 Biennale of Sydney in Sydney, Australia, and the 1997 UAAC conference in Vancouver. A book of his writings titled *Everything is Relevant: Writings on Art and Life 1991–2018* was published in 2020 by Concordia University Press.

Since the mid-1990s, Lum has worked on numerous major permanent public art commissions including for the cities of Vienna, Rotterdam, St. Louis, Leiden, Utrecht, Toronto, and Vancouver.

He was Project Manager for the seminal exhibition, *The Short Century: Independence and Liberation Movements in Africa, 1945–1994.*

Lum co-curated *Shanghai Modern: 1919–1945; Sharjah Biennial 7, Sharjah, United Arab Emirates* and *Monument Lab: Creative Speculations for Philadelphia.*

Lum is the Co-Founder and Senior Curatorial Advisor to Monument Lab, a public art and history collective founded in Philadelphia.

Robin Alex McDonald lives and works on Robinson-Huron Treaty territory, the traditional territory of the Anishnaabeg people and, specifically, the Nipissing First Nation. Robin teaches in the Department of Fine and Performing Arts at Nipissing University as well as the Liberal Arts Department at OCAD University. They are also an independent curator and arts writer. Their research explores representations of depression in queer contemporary art.

Karin Michalski works as artist, film and video art curator and lecturer in Berlin. With her films and videos such as *The Alphabet of Feeling Bad* (2014, text-based video projection), *The Alphabet of Feeling Bad* (2012), *Working on it* (2008, Co-Director: Sabian Baumann), *Monika M.* (2004), *Pashke and Sofia* (2003) she has been invited to numerous festivals and exhibitions. Since 2001 she has been organizing the queer-feminist Film and Video Art Program series clipclub (in collaboration with Renate Lorenz) and she works as film and video art curator, creating programs for art institutions, festivals, and conferences. In 2016 she co-edited the artist edition *An Unhappy Archive*, Edition Fink, Zurich, and in 2015 the book *I is for Impasse, Affektive Queerverbindungen in Theorie_Aktivismus_Kunst*, bbooks, Berlin, as well as in 2011 the fanzine FEELING BAD—queer pleasures, art & politics. She also works as lecturer at art academies and universities.

José Esteban Muñoz was a writer and scholar who taught at and served as chair of the department of Performance Studies at the Tisch School of the Arts, New York University.

Sabrina Reed is Professor of English in the Department of English, Languages, and Cultures at Mount Royal University in Calgary, where she has divided her career between teaching and administrative roles. She obtained her Ph.D. in Canadian Literature from the University of Toronto in 1988. Sabrina is interested in illness narratives and especially in portrayals of mental illnesses and other conditions that do not have obvious physiological causes. She takes an interdisciplinary approach which combines medical and lay perspectives. She is currently working on a monograph on Miriam Toews.

Vivek Shraya is an artist whose body of work crosses the boundaries of music, literature, visual art, theater, and film. Her best-selling book *I'm Afraid of Men* was heralded by *Vanity Fair* as "cultural rocket fuel," and her album *PartTime Woman* was nominated for the Polaris Music Prize.

She is also the founder of the publishing imprint VS. Books. A six-time Lambda Literary Award finalist, Vivek was a Pride Toronto Grand Marshal and was featured on The Globe and Mail's Best Dressed list. She is a director on the board of the Tegan and Sara Foundation, an Assistant Professor of Creative Writing at the University of Calgary, and is currently adapting her debut play, *How To Fail As A Popstar*, into a television pilot script with the support of CBC.

John Streamas received his Ph.D. in American Culture Studies from Bowling Green State University after graduating from Syracuse University's program in creative writing, where his advisors were George P. Elliott and Raymond Carver. An immigrant biracial Asian American and first-generation college student, he has researched histories and cultures of wartime Japanese American incarceration and of American communities of color generally. He has published on racial politics in film and literature, and his special interest in the politics of racialized time and space has materialized in published essays on nonlinear temporalities in writers of color and the ethics of barbed wire. Aside from scholarly work, Streamas has also published fiction, poetry, and personal essays. His manuscript in progress examines time in cultures of color. Currently he is an Associate Professor of comparative ethnic studies in the School of Languages, Cultures, and Race at Washington State University.

Zoë Brigley Thompson is Assistant Professor at the Ohio State University. She has a B.A. in Creative Writing, a M.A. in Gender and Literature, and a Ph.D. in Comparative Literary Studies all from University of Warwick, England. She won an Eric Gregory Award for the best British poets under 30 and was longlisted for the Dylan Thomas Prize for the best international writers under 40. She has published three collections of poetry *The Secret* (2007), *Conquest* (2012), and *Hand & Skull* (2019), all of which were Poetry Book Society Recommendations. Her nonfiction essays *Notes from a Swing State* were published in 2019, and she edited the Routledge volume *Feminism, Literature, and Rape Narratives* (2010) with Sorcha Gunne. She has published peer-review essays in *Gender and Education, The Journal of Gender Studies, Feminist Media Studiesm Feminist Formations,* and *Contemporary Women's Writing*. She is currently editing *The Bloomsbury Companion to Contemporary Poetry in Ireland and the UK.*

Fan Wu believes himself a nomadic aether-object you can beam into at will. His academic-creative practice is moving toward translation, adaptation, receptivity, and non-striving. He hosts sympedagogical workshops in collaboration with arts institutions in Toronto, including Art Metropole, Trinity Square Video, and Mercer Union. You can find and read his writing online at baest journal, Aisle 4, Koffler Digital, MICE Magazine, and C Magazine.

CHAPTER 1

Re/Imagining Depression

Robin Alex McDonald and Julie Hollenbach

Re/Imagining Depression: Creative Approaches to "Feeling Bad" began with the troubling awareness that a preoccupation with identifiable symptoms, a privileging of diagnoses, and attention to medications had come to dominate how we—the editors, two queer art historians, close friends, and co-conspirators—spoke to one another about our experiences of depression, loss, and living. As writers and arts workers with penchants for poetics and whimsy, our inabilities to untether our heavy feelings and our slow bodies from the biomedical distressed us, not least because it suggested that we were losing our grip on the very forms of creativity and imagination that normally buoyed us. When we encountered Ann Cvetkovich's book, *Depression: A Public Feeling*, when it was first published in 2012, its critique of the pathologizing, homogenizing, and universalizing nature of medical discourses on depression and trauma resonated with us. We were both familiar with Cvetkovich's work before

R. A. McDonald (✉)
Fine and Performing Arts, Nipissing University, North Bay, ON, Canada

J. Hollenbach
NSCAD University, Halifax, NS, Canada
e-mail: jhollenbach@nscad.ca

J. Hollenbach and R. A. McDonald (eds.), *Re/Imagining Depression*,
https://doi.org/10.1007/978-3-030-80554-8_1

this book; Julie had leant Robin her copy of Cvetkovich's *An Archive of Feelings: Trauma, Sexuality, and Lesbian Public Cultures* (2003) soon after meeting in grad school, and we bonded over the way the book breathed new life into academic writing for us. When Cvetkovich's transition from trauma to depression in 2012 brought her work more in line with Julie's research on craft and Robin's research on depression, our conversations around affect and public feelings were reignited.

In *Depression*, Cvetkovich seeks to understand depression as intimately embedded in the textures of everyday life and its structures. Following Raymond Williams, Cvetkovich posits depression simultaneously as a "structure of feeling," an affective dimension of sociopolitical life shaped by neoliberal capitalism, colonialism, White supremacy, and patriarchy, as well as an "ordinary affect" that resides in the nooks and crannies of the quotidian (Williams 1977; Cvetkovich 2012, pp. 11, 13). This effort to reframe depression as a political feeling goes hand-in-hand with Cvetkovich's call to "depathologize negative feelings" and her subsequent claim that "accounts of depression require new ways of talking about affective states and making them publicly significant" (2012, pp. 2, 157–158). Cvetkovich's preferred term, "feeling bad," initiates some of this work because "its colloquial blandness is an invitation to further elaboration, which can consist in an anecdote," as well as, we add, in the types of personal accounts and theoretical musings contained within this anthology (pp. 157–158).

Tracing the Ascendency of Psychiatric Discourses

That heavy and amorphous cluster of emotions, behaviors, and embodiments, which today "gets called depression," has been referred to by many other names: from black bile and melancholy to an "imagined sun, bright and black at the same time" and a "noonday demon" (Cvetkovich 2012, p. 25; Kristeva 1989; Solomon 2001). Although for well over a century Western psychiatric and medical discourses have exerted a stranglehold on how we talk—and how we *can* talk—about depression, creative sites such as literature, poetry, theory, performance, visual art, and film have historically offered, and continue to offer, new languages for speaking about "bad feelings." Before discussing how these sites may contribute to a multiplication of discourse on depression and experiences of "feeling bad," we want to briefly consider how, exactly, depression came to be so heavily pathologized in the contemporary moment.

Though the history we trace here is, necessarily, an incomplete one, we hope that it might offer some sense of the recentness of this development, and so also suggest the impermanence of this episteme.

As French cultural critic Michel Foucault makes clear in *The Birth of the Clinic*, the introduction of modern medicine instituted an epistemological rupture that generated new discourses of knowledge about the body through observation and diagnosis (Foucault 1975). As early as 1840, statistical information about madness, including its rates and locations, has been collected and cataloged in the United States (APA website, History of the *DSM*). In 1921, the American Medico-Psychological Association (later renamed the American Psychiatric Association, hereafter referred to as the APA) and the New York Academy of Medicine co-created a "nationally acceptable psychiatric classification" that was published within the first edition of the American Medical Association's Standard Classified Nomenclature of Disease (APA 2009). Approximately thirty years later, the APA Committee on Nomenclature and Statistics developed the first edition of the *Diagnostic and Statistical Manual of Mental Disorders* (hereafter referred to as the *DSM*) using a variant of the World Health Organization's sixth edition of the *International Classification of Diseases* (*ICD*) (APA website, History of the *DSM*). This version of the *DSM* placed considerable emphasis on the social and environmental causes of disorders, referred to as "reactions;" thus, the entry on "Depressive Reaction" described depression as "precipitated by a current situation" and tied depression to loss, failure, and guilt (Horwitz 2014, pp. 2–3). However, when the *DSM* was revised in 1968, the *DSM-II* shifted emphasis from the depressive's environment to the depressive's own psyche. Referred to as "Depressive Neurosis," the disorder was said to be "manifested by an excessive reaction of depression due to an internal conflict or to an identifiable event such as the loss of a love object or cherished possession" (Horwitz 2014, pp. 2–3). Thus, the cause of depression was reframed from the individual's environment to the individual's *reaction* to that environment, effectively relocating the origin of the affect within the individual and the personal.

As the pharmaceutical treatment of mental disorders grew during the late twentieth century, the *DSM* once again shifted from "perfunctory definitions" to "precise, symptom-based classifications" (Kramer 1993; Healy 2004; Kirsch 2009). In 1975, the *DSM-III* expanded from 182 diagnoses to 265, evidencing the emergence of what Jennifer Radden has termed "drug cartography," that is, a shift in which diagnostic criteria went from being primarily based on observed symptoms to being based on what a particular pharmaceutical medication (supposedly) alleviates (2003, p. 38). Marie Allitt's chapter in this volume, "'Titled Things:' Materiality and Reification in Antidepressant Narratives," thinks critically about this "drug cartography" and its implications for antidepressant users, diverging from critiques of the mass-prescribing of these medications to instead focus on "the relationship between patient and prescription." (Allit, this volume.) Here, Allitt looks to the life writing of Lauren Slater and Elizabeth Wurtzel to think about antidepressant medications in relation to both biomedical discourses, and the corporeal rituals of ingestion and incorporation, in order to argue that pills and capsules validate, visualize, and reify the abstract concept of "mental illness."

Since its initial publication in 1952, the *DSM* has undergone several further updates, including the *DSM-III-R* in 1987, the *DSM-IV* in 1994, and finally the *DSM-V,* which was published in 2013. Within the most recent edition of the *DSM-V,* which was last updated in 2015, the section on "Depressive Disorders" spans a collection of eight disorders that includes Disruptive Mood Dysregulation Disorder; Major Depressive Disorder; Persistent Depressive Disorder (Dysthymia); Premenstrual Dysphoric Disorder; Substance/Medication-Induced Depressive Disorder; Depressive Disorder Due to Another Medical Condition; Other Specified Depressive Disorder; Unspecified Depressive Disorder. While the introduction of these subsets of depressive disorders *appears* to offer more discourses for speaking about depression, the newly available terms also serve to produce new sites of regulation, control, and subject formation (Foucault 1976 [1978, p. 137]).

This present era of psychiatry and the pathologization of bad feelings eclipses many forms of thinking about "feeling bad" that came before it, including Ancient Greek discourses of melancholy and black bile or Early Christian monks' concept of acedia. It also overshadows the history of the "blue ecological aesthetic" of medieval literature, as Jes Battis discusses in his chapter, "Blue Histories: Thinking With Sadness in the Middle Ages," (Joy 2013, p. 215 cited by Battis, this volume), as well as what Zoe Brigley Thompson, following Julia Kristeva, identifies as *ekstasis*—a form of epiphanic metaphysicality that Thompson suggests is embodied in the figure of the angel, as rendered by Rainer Maria Rilke (Kristeva 1989 cited by Thompson, this volume). Perhaps even more acutely, the contemporary era of psychiatric discourses also obfuscates colonial and imperial histories of enslavement and displacement, cultural and literal genocides, and ongoing occupations of land, which, as many Critical Race scholars have pointed out, continue to impact the emotional, psychological, and embodied lives of Black people, Indigenous people, and other people of color (Cheng 2001; Eng and Han 2003; Gilroy 2005). In their respective chapters, "Feeling Brown Feeling Down: Latina Affect, The Performativity of Race, and the Depressive Position" and "Not Down but Different: Depression in the Shadow of the Black Dog," José Esteban Muñoz and John Streamas each discuss the "material contingencies" of these ongoing processes, demonstrating the ways in which they constitute a pervasive sense of "brownness" that cannot be remedied through neoliberal "diversity" initiatives (Muñoz; Streamas, this volume).

"Creative" Approaches

In referring to the approaches in this book as "creative," we follow Ann Cvetkovich's description of depression "as blockage or impasse or being stuck," whose "cure might lie in forms of flexibility or creativity" (Cvetkovich, p. 21). While we see depression itself as an experience of "being stuck," we also suggest that much of the contemporary writing on depression has been "stuck" in Western psychiatric discourses, "stuck" in the memoir genre, "stuck" in Whiteness, and "stuck" on the unit of the individual. This anthology also seeks to unstick scholarship on depression from the field's normatively-presumed subject: the White cisgender woman. As many scholars have noted, depression is a feminized diagnosis, much more likely to be applied to women than men (Jack 1991; Stoppard 2000; Maracek 2006; Lafrance 2009). However, as Muñoz observes, "the topic of depression has not often been discussed in relation to the question of racial formations in critical theory" (Munoz 2006, reprinted in this volume). Nyasha Junior similarly points out in her chapter, "Don't We Hurt Like You? Examining the Lack of Portrayals of African American Women and Mental Health," originally published in *Bitch Magazine*'s Summer 2015 issue, that the experience of depression in Black women is often denied, reframed, or misdiagnosed due to the normalization of Black women's pain (Junior, this volume). While it is not our intention (nor, we assume, the intentions of this anthology's contributors) to pathologize the emotional effects of racism and colonialism by labelling them as "depression," we do hope that by critiquing depression as a narrowly-applied biomedical discursive formation we might make space for other conceptualizations of "feeling bad" that pay closer attention to race and other intersections of identity.

Literature and Language

Thankfully, as Cvetkovich points out, despite the current hegemony of the biomedical model, "there are other archives besides the specific-turned-universal of medical perspectives (or the Western humanist tradition of melancholy)" (2012, p. 160). In turning away from psychology and medicine and toward the arts and humanities, we re-orient this anthology toward the generative potentials of poetry, fiction, and the image. Within these creative sites, metaphor, symbolism, and abstraction muddy and complicate understandings of depression, rather than to clarify or refine them. In her chapter, "Teaching/Depression as a Queer Theory for Living," for example, Alyson Hoy explains how renowned queer theorist Eve Kosofsky Sedgwick "adopts an ancient Japanese poetic form called *haibun*, which mixes prose with haiku." Hoy explains that when Sedgwick

> weaves haiku into her prose the white space between lines, between poetry and prose, become the empty spaces through which many meanings pass. This is, for Sedgwick, reparation writ large: the use of a multiplicity of perspectives to replace dualistic thinking with a more open epistemology, and the writing of a text that, in privileging processes and practices of realization and understanding, prompts other ways of thinking about illness. (Hoy, this volume)

Hoy suggests that Sedgwick's use of *haibun* constitutes a "queer genre," one that revels in complexities and multiplicities, one that can sustain the messiness and fragmentedness of thought—and of life—and Sedgwick confirms this reading in her own observation of the "power" of enjambment as well as the "transfigurative (i.e. misrecognition-creating) potential of any art" (Sedgwick 1987, pp. 114, 138 [n6]). Similarly, in "On Being Ill," Virginia Woolf argues that "in illness words seem to possess a mystic quality. We grasp what is beyond their surface meaning, gather instinctively this, that, and the other – a sound, a color, here a stress, there a pause[…]" (1930, p. 21). For Woolf, illness (and it is clear that much of Woolf's experiences of illness would today be classified as *mental* illness) encourages readers to encounter text primarily through the senses rather than the intellect, and with an openness to incomprehensibility that allows for a unique appreciation of the obscure and the obtuse.

Depression has found a suitable home in writing for several decades now, particularly in the genre of memoir, where the form of the "autopathography" "restores the person ignored or canceled out in the medical enterprise[…], places that person at the very center […and] gives that ill person a voice" (Hawkins 1999, p. 12) Sabrina Reed's chapter, "Being Sita," considers Gayathri Ramprasad's memoir, *Shadows in the Sun: Healing from Depression and Finding the Light Within* (2014), through the lens of Carl Elliott's theories on how alienation may cause or exacerbate depression. In doing so, Reed elucidates how the genre of memoir continues to serve as a valuable resource for validating personal experience and rendering the personal political.

Reed demonstrates how the depression memoir also effectively becomes company for Raprasad; the salve for the alienation of depression. In the void of depression, the memoir provides a horizon, a sense of perspective, a direction that is up and out from the avalanche of discordant and numb feeling. Similarly, in francesca ekwuyasi's chapter, "i want to be a seashell, i want to be a mold, i want to be a spirit," ekwuyasi crafts her own version of a depression-memoir, in which she reflects on the cruel juxtaposition between her proclivity for words and the difficulty of writing when depressed; how following words can be a "quixotic" and pleasurable quest sometimes, and a heavy and cumbersome burden others.

Art and the Visual

Woolf seems to agree with ekwuyasi, arguing that any literary description of illness is always already hindered by "the poverty of language" (Woolf 1930). Perhaps this is why Julia Kristeva instead champions not the writer but the artist as "melancholy's most intimate witness and the fiercest fighter against the symbolic abdication enveloping him" (Woolf 1930; Kristeva 1987). For Kristeva:

> the depressed person, overwhelmed by sadness[…], suffers from a paralysis of symbolic activity. In effect, language fails to substitute for what has been lost at the level of the psyche. The loss of loved ones, the loss of ideals, the loss of pasts: as the depressed person loses all interest in the surrounding world, in language itself, psychic energy shifts to a more

> primitive mode of functioning, to a maternal, drive-oriented form of experience. In short, depression produces a trauma of symbolic identification, a trauma that unleashes the power of semiotic energy. (Elliot summarizing Kristeva 2016, n.p.)

For Kristeva, if Melanie Klein's "depressive position" occurs as a result of the subject's entrance into the father's realm of language and culture, then engagements with signs and symbols may offer a kind of ***return*** to the original state of unity with the mother, for which the depressed person unconsciously longs (Klein 1935; Kristeva 1989). Thus for Kristeva, art—in all of its various, disparate, wonderful forms—holds onto the possibility for "remaining optimistic within this depressive moment" (1998, p. 6). In this anthology, Pansee Atta's interview with Vivek Shraya, Sima Godfrey's dialogue with Ken Lum, and José Esteban Muñoz's chapter on the work of Nao Bustamante and Bas Jan Ader, each offer compelling evidence for the unique abilities of visual and performance art to communicate gestures, expressions, and refusals which language cannot speak. However, these authors contradict Kristeva's belief in art's inherent optimism; Lum, for example, states that his "work was never about redemption, but what was real. It was always concerned with facing up to the real and then asking the question: and then what?" (Lum, this volume).

An Anthology, an Altar, an Archive

It feels poignant that this book will be published amidst the backdrop of the COVID-19 pandemic, a time in which reported rates of depression and other mental health issues are estimated to have tripled (Ettman et al. 2020). In the anthology's final two essays, "Bird Says the Sound of Rewind" by Hamish Ballantyne and Fan Wu and "The present is what we are doing together" by Feel Tank Chicago, the authors reflect directly on how the events of 2020 (including but not limited to the pandemic, Black Lives Matter protests against police brutality and systemic anti-Blackness, and the United States presidential election) have transformed the affective landscape of our daily lives. The conditions of everyday life for many people, even those of relative socioeconomic privilege, now mirror the conditions of depressive episodes: physical and social isolation, a lack of optimism about the future, emotional unpredictability and dysregulation, and a tendency toward escapisms and dissociation. This collective trauma has come to infiltrate even the most banal elements of everyday life, has suspended hope, has put our world's existing inequities into a pressure cooker. In these moments, it is difficult to know where to start, where to begin, or how to move forward.

Cvetkovich uses the term "bibliographic altar" to describe a "set of sources that has become precious" (Cvetkovich and Wilkerson 2016, p. 498). In an interview with disability studies scholar Abby Wilkerson, Cvetkovich shares photos of these altars, manifested as physical assemblages of academic books, graphic novels, compact discs (including Le Tigre's *This Island* from 2004 and Kiki and Herb's *Will Die for You* from 2005), mugs, photographs, loose papers, bright pink squirrel-like creatures created by craft-artist Allyson Mitchell, half-melted candles, and a statue of the Virgin of Guadalupe. Reminiscent of Tracey Emin's 1998 installation *My Bed*, in which Emin relocated her bed—the scene of an extensive depressive episode—replete with empty vodka bottles, condoms, cigarette butts, and stained bedsheets into the gallery space, these altars reveal how the objects that cohere around depressed bodies shed light on both the experience of depression and strategies for survival. Indeed, Cvetkovich refers to the books and music that she lays upon her altars as having "saved [her] life and helped [her] keep writing" (Cvetkovich and Wilkerson 2016, p. 498). Following Cvetkovich, we like to think of this anthology as its own kind of altar, which assembles texts that are precious to their authors, that have become precious to us as editors, and that we hope may become precious to readers, too.

We begin the anthology with Ann Cvetkovich and Karin Michalski's collaborative project, *The Alphabet of Feeling Bad* (2012) in order to signal our debt to Cvetkovich's thinking around politics and affect, but also in the hopes of providing the reader with a sort of "toolkit" for approaching the rest of the book. In their project, Cvetkovich and Michalski generate an encyclopedia of emotion in which "the dialectic of hope and despair that underlies 'The Alphabet's' effort to name bad feelings" also serves to produce new forms of "collectivity and survival" (Cvetkovich, this volume). It is our hope (and also our despair) that this toolkit, and everything that follows it, may offer a means of thinking about and through the quagmire of our collective present.

References

APA. 2009. *DSM* History. Retrieved 25 July 2021. http://www.psychiatry.org/practice/dsm/dsm-history-of-the-manual.

Cheng, Anne. 2001. *The Melancholy of Race*. New York: Oxford University Press.

Cvetkovich, Ann. 2003. *An Archive of Feeling: Trauma, Sexuality, and Lesbian Public Cutures*. Durham: Duke University Press.

———. 2012. *Depression: A Public Feeling*. Durham: Duke University Press.

Cvetkovich, Ann, and Abby Wilkerson. 2016. Disability and *Depression. Bioethical Inquiry* 13: 497–503.

Elliot, Anthony. 2016. *Identity Troubles: An Introduction*. Oxon and New York: Routledge.

Eng, David, and Shin-Hee Han. 2003. A Dialogue on Racial Melancholia. In *Loss: The Politics of Mourning*, ed. David Eng and David Kazanjian, 343–371. Berkeley: University of California Press.

Ettman, Catherine, Salma M. Abdalla, Gregory H. Cohen, Laura Sampson, Patrick M. Vivier, and Sandro Galea. 2020. Prevalence of Depression Symptoms in US Adults Before and During the COVID-19 Pandemic. *JAMA Network Open* 3 (9): np.

Foucault, Michel. 1975. *The Birth of the Clinic. An Archaeology of Medical Perception*. New York: Vintage Books.

———. 1976. *History of Sexuality. Volume 1: The Will to Knowledge*, trans. Robert Hurley. New York: Pantheon Books.

Gilroy, Paul. 2005. *Postcolonial Melancholia*. New York: Columbia University Press.

Hawkins, Anne Hunsaker. 1999. *Reconstructing Illness: Studies in Pathography*. West Lafayette: Purdue Research Foundation.

Healy, David. 2004. *Let Them Eat Prozac: The Unhealthy Relationship Between the Pharmaceutical Industry and Depression*. New York, NY: New York University Press.

Horwitz, Allan V. 2014. DSM-I and DSM-II. In *The Encyclopedia of Clinical Psychology*, 1st ed., ed. Robin L. Cautin and Scott O. Lilienfeld. Wiley.

Jack, Dana C. 1991. *Silencing the Self: Women and Depression*. Harvard University Press.

Joy, Eileen. 2013. Blue. In *Prismatic Ecology: Ecotheory Beyond Green*, ed. Jeffrey Jerome Cohen, 213–232. Minneapolis: University of Minnesota Press.

Kirsch, Irving. 2009. *The Emperor's New Drugs: Exploding the Antidepressant Myth*. London: Random House Books.

Klein, Melanie. 1935. A Contribution to the Psychogenesis of Manic-Depressive States. *International Journal of PsychoAnalysis* 16: 145–174.

Kramer, Peter D. 1993. *Listening to Prozac*. New York, NY: Viking Press.

Kristeva, Julia. 1987. On the Melancholy Imaginary. In *Discourse in Psychoanalysis and Literature*, ed. Schlomith Rimmon-Kenan. London: Routledge.

———. 1989. *Black Sun: Depression and Melancholia*, trans. Leon S. Roudiez. New York: Columbia University Press.

———. 1998. Dialogue with Julia Kristeva. *Parallax* 4 (3).

Lafrance, Michelle. 2009. *Women and Depression: Recovery and Resistance*. Sussex and New York: Routledge.

Marecek, J. 2006. Social Suffering, Gender, and Women's Depression. In *Women and Depression: A Handbook for the Social, Behavioral, and Biomedical Sciences*, ed. C.L.M. Keyes and S.H. Goodman, 283–308. Cambridge University Press.

Muñoz, José Esteban. 2006. Feeling Brown, Feeling Down: Latina Affect, the Performativity of Race, and the Depressive Position. *Signs* 31 (3). New Feminist Theories of Visual Culture, 675–688

Radden, Jennifer. 2003. Is This Dame Melancholy?: Equating Today's Depression and Past Melancholia. *Philosophy, Psychiatry, & Psychology* 10 (1): 37–52.

Sedgwick, Eve Kosofsky. 1987. A Poem is Being Written. *Representations* 17 Special Issue: The Cultural Display of the Body: 110–143.

Solomon, Andrew. 2001. *The Noonday Demon*. New York: Scribner.

Stoppard, Janet M. 2000. *Understanding Depression: Feminist Social Constructionist Approaches*. London and New York: Routledge.

Williams, Raymond. 1977. Structures of Feeling. In *Marxism and Literature*, 128–225. New York: Oxford University Press.

Woolf, Virginia. 1930. *On Being Ill*. London: Hogarth Press.

CHAPTER 2

The Alphabet of Feeling Bad Now

Ann Cvetkovich and Karin Michalski

When Karin Michalski invited me to join her for a one-day film shoot in Berlin in April 2012 with the aim of turning a list of feeling words into a lecture-performance for an installation video called *The Alphabet of Feeling Bad*, I had no idea that the project would have such an extensive life across exhibitions, lectures, print publications, and even an audio recording. My collaboration with Michalski was a creative gift that has led to many inspiring events, especially in Europe (see list at the close of this chapter). Having theories about political depression and queer affect turned into an art project has made them not only more accessible but more exciting.

As time passes, *The Alphabet of Feeling Bad* also functions as an archive of a certain moment in queer affect theory, especially the turn to negative affect in concepts such as Sara Ahmed's *killjoy*, Lauren Berlant's

The correction of this chapter can be found under https://doi.org/10.1007/978-3-030-80554-8_16

A. Cvetkovich (✉)
Carleton University, Ottawa, ON, Canada
e-mail: anncvetkovich@cunet.carleton.ca

K. Michalski
Berlin, Germany
e-mail: contact@karinmichalski.de

J. Hollenbach and R. A. McDonald (eds.), *Re/Imagining Depression*,
https://doi.org/10.1007/978-3-030-80554-8_2

cruel optimism and *slow death*, Heather Love's *feeling backward,* José Muñoz's *feeling brown* and *cruising utopia*—and my collective participation in Feel Tank's coinage of the term *political depression* (Ahmed 2010; Berlant 2011; Love 2007; Muñoz 2000, 2009). Indeed, the screening of *The Alphabet* as part of "unhappy archive" exhibitions included a display of their books and others in the gallery space so as to introduce viewers to this body of work. Clustered together, we constitute a loose school of thinking about bad feelings that resists the vocabulary of clinical psychology and medical diagnosis.

On the occasion of text version of *The Alphabet*'s publication here, close to ten years after its original conception, one of the questions that emerges is whether feeling bad feels the same way now as it did then. Are we still feeling bad? And if so, are there new vocabularies of bad feeling?

Given the current political climate, the answer to the first question would seem to be an emphatic yes. The election of Donald Trump and many other reactionary demagogic leaders intent on destroying public culture and the welfare state, anti-immigration backlash everywhere, climate change and environmental disaster, anti-Black violence, and failed and repressed revolutions are just a few of the developments that have us reeling—and we must now add to that list the covid-19 pandemic. The dialectic of hope and despair that underlies *The Alphabet*'s effort to name bad feelings as a way of also producing collectivity and survival remains pertinent—and perhaps explains its persistent life. But I also find myself experiencing new levels of panic, urgency, and helplessness and regularly find others in the same state. I would be wary of shuttling these new feelings into the homogenous category of negative affect, but the entanglement or dialectic of hope and despair, and positive and negative feelings of many kinds, is constant. As is the value of describing what's happening not just in terms of external political situations but also in terms of the moods and affects they create, which are a more amorphous fusion of the external and internal, the individual and the collective. I have also found useful our fellow traveler Debbie Gould's thinking about "not knowing" as an important affective response to the dangerously black and white thinking of political leaders and other "experts."

I thus like to think that *The Alphabet* as a project remains relevant—even if the vocabularies change—especially since it was intended as an invitation to add new words for present conditions and is a format designed to be flexible and adaptable to new circumstances. Nonetheless, I think the category of *(political) depression* and/or *feeling bad* remains relevant, especially given the ongoing epidemic of depression and anxiety—and the problematic medicalization of these feeling states—in the worlds I inhabit. Of late, I find particularly valuable practices and vocabularies of care activisms, which provide answers to the perennial question of "what is to be done?" that are very practical and affectively driven. Disability activists, Indigenous feminists, queer and trans people of color, and others are creating new ways of thinking about how we can support one another in the face of destruction and the despair it generates. This anthology, for example, participates in the turn to mad studies and critical disability studies that has generated new ways of thinking about mental health. I'm happy to think that *The Alphabet of Feeling Bad* might continue to be a resource for survival.

A is for Anxiety and for Alienation.
A is also for Acedia, a medieval word
for the lethargy of spiritual despair.

B is for Backward,
as in Feeling Backward.
Or left out or like a misfit.
Feeling Backward can also mean looking to the
past to make connections with people from
other times who might have been queer and who can
become our fellow travelers.

C is for Capitalism,
as in "You might be suffering from Capitalism."
But saying that capitalism is the problem
doesn't always help me get up in the morning.

D is for Depression,
for Despair,
for Doubt,
for Disappointment
and for Dread.

E is for the Everyday
because feeling bad is a very ordinary
and Everyday experience.

F is for Failure,
which is not always a bad thing since the Failure to be
normal can be good.

F is also for Feeling Bad.
The Alphabet of Feeling Bad is about creating
new vocabularies but sometimes very simple
statements like "I feel bad" are the best way to
describe our feelings.

G is for Grief.
I don't think that needs an explanation.

H is for Happiness.
Happiness is a tricky term.
Because the things that are supposed to make us
happy often don't succeed in doing so.
It's important to question what counts as Happiness
and make room for feelings of Unhappiness that
express the desire for a different kind of world.

H is also for Hopelessness,
which is one of the deadliest forms of feeling bad.
Depression comes from the Hopelessness of
being unable to imagine a future.
The cultivation of Hope is an important struggle
especially because there are so many
good reasons to lose Hope.

I is for Impasse.
I often feel like I don't know what to do
or like I'm stuck.
Being at an Impasse is not always a bad thing.
Sometimes it's important to dwell in the space of not
knowing what to do.

J is for Jaded and for Jealousy.
Jealousy can be a political disappointment,
the failure of feminist dreams of sisterhood.
We want to learn to accept Jealousy as
part of collective life.

K is for Killjoy.
Feminists are often called Killjoys.
The Killjoy is the person who resents other

people's pleasure or remains stubbornly
unhappy in the midst of their joy.
Sometimes it's important to be the Killjoy – to say
"Fuck you – I am not feeling it.
Your version of happiness is really
problematic for me."

L is for Loneliness.
Is it possible to share the feeling of being
lonely or alone as a way to make new forms
of collectivity?

M is for Melancholy
and also for Melodrama.
I like Melodrama because it often provides a public
forum for women who are feeling bad.

N is for Normalcy,
which we want to challenge.
We want to embrace feelings that are
considered abnormal.

N is also for Numbness.
Sometimes feeling bad means feeling numb because
we feel like we don't have any
feelings when there is no public space for them.
But Numbness is a feeling too.
And feeling numb can protect us from
feeling too much.

O is for Occupy,
which has become the name for
a political movement.
But sometimes we are so distracted,
or pre-occupied, by feeling bad
that we don't have time for politics.
How can we bring together the emotional
and political meanings of Occupy?
How can paying attention to our feelings
become part of our political movements?

P is for Precarity,
a word that has been used to describe
those who fall outside of material

and economic systems of support.
Precarity could also describe
how feeling bad puts many people,
even those who have material privilege,
in a state of emotional Precarity.

P is for Passivity,
which is another feeling that shouldn't be
easily dismissed.
We are often told that in order to be good activists we
have to get rid of our Passivity.
What if radical Passivity were also a way to
get things done?

P is also for Public Feelings,
the name of the group I've been working
with for some time.
Our goal is to pay attention to feelings as a shared
experience not a private or individual one.
We dream of being able to have our
feelings together in order to feel a little less lonely
and more public.

Q is for Queer, of course.
And for the idea that there is no feeling
that is too Queer.
Let's have more words for feelings that seem
strange or Queer!

R is for Rage.
R is for Revolution.
And R is for Respite.
For the desire to take a break to have some time out
to stop when you are burned out.
There is so much pressure to keep up and to
keep moving and sometimes we just need
to slow down.

S is for Slow Death.
Slow Death describes how the daily routines
of living with structural inequalities,
and the things we are attached to, can wear us out.

S is also for Shame,
which is a very important queer feeling.

T is for Trauma.

U is for Utopia.
In my version of Utopia,
there is plenty of room for bad feelings.

V is for Vulnerability,
which is another feeling that has
gotten a bad reputation.
I want to welcome Vulnerability as the
way in which we make ourselves open to ourselves
and to others.
Vulnerability can be the
foundation for connection.

W is for Weariness
and for the War on Worries.
Instead of the War on Terrorism, let's have the War on
Worries in which we battle against the demons that
make us feel bad and wage war on the
sensations of racism, sexism and homophobia.

X is for Extreme as in Extreme feelings.
X is also for Exhaustion.

Y is for Yawn and also for Yell,
which are two different ways
of expressing feelings.

And Z is for Zest.
Zest is energy, vitality, life force.
We want to cultivate Zest including the energy
of feeling bad.

References

Ahmed, Sara. 2010. *The Promise of Happiness*. Durham: Duke University Press.

Berlant, Lauren. 2011. *Cruel Optimism*. Durham: Duke University Press.

Love, Heather. 2007. *Feeling Backward: Loss and the Politics of Queer History.*

Muñoz, José Esteban. 2000. Feeling Brown: Ethnicity and Affect in Ricardo Bracho's The Sweetest Hangover (and Other STDs). *Theatre Journal* 52 (1): 67–79.

———. 2009. *Cruising Utopia: The Then and There of Queer Futurity.* New York: New York University Press.

The Alphabet of Feeling Bad

Publications

Baumann, Sabian, and Karin Michalski. 2016. *An Unhappy Archive*. Zurich: Edition Fink [Artist book with LP recording].

Cvetkovich, Ann. 2014. Writing with *The Alphabet of Feeling Bad*. In *Walking Beside: Challenging the Role of Emotions in Normalization*, ed. Eva Söderberg and Sara Nyhlén, 37–51. Forum for Gender Studies Working Papers. Sundsvall: Mid Sweden University.

———. 2019. *The Alphabet of Feeling Bad*: Environmental Installation Arts and Sensory Publics. In *Public Spheres of Resonance: Constellations of Affect and Language*, ed. Anne Flieg and Christian von Scheve, 151–172. New York: Routledge.

Hauser, Fanny, and Victor Neumann. (Eds.). 2021. *Wicked Little Town*. Berlin: Archive Books.

von Bose, Käthe, Ulrike Klöppel, Katrin Köppert, Karin Michalski, and Pat Treusch. 2015. *I is for Impasse: Affecktiv Queerverbindungen in Theorie_Aktivismus_Kunst*. Berlin: b-books.

Galleries, Exhibitions, and Websites

Karin Michalski http://www.karinmichalski.de.

2012

A Burnt-Out Case, nGbK Gallery. Berlin, Germany. https://archiv.ngbk.de/en/projekte/a-burnt-out-case/.

Axe Grinding Workshop. Tate Modern, London. http://www.tate.org.uk/whats-on/tate-modern/conference/axe-grinding-workshop.

PREVIEW Berlin Art Fair. http://www.previewberlin.de/.

Tender Buttons, Gallery September. Berlin, Germany. http://www.september-berlin.com/exhibition/review/73/en.

2013

Les Complices. Zurich, Switzerland. http://www.lescomplices.ch/recollect/the-alphabet-of-feeling-bad/the-alphabet-of-feeling-bad/.
Visualising Affect. Lewisham Arthouse, London, England. http://visualisingaffect.weebly.com; http://www.lewishamarthouse.org.uk.

2014

An Unhappy Archive. Badischer Kunstverein, Karlsruhe, Germany. http://www.badischer-kunstverein.de/index.php?Direction=Programm&Detail=552.
Counterparts. Institute for Contemporary Art and Ideas, Gothenburg, Sweden. http://www.icia.se/en/exhibition/counterparts/.
Station 21, Art Space. Zurich, Switzerland. http://www.station21.ch/.
Words Needed. *Umeå* European *Capital* of *Culture 2014*. Sweden. http://umea2014.se/en/event/words-needed/.

2015

Get Well Soon! Cultural Center, Potsdam, Germany. www.getwellsoonexhibition.tumblr.com.

2017

Mic Drop, Exhibition, & Performance Festival. Innsbruck, Austria. https://micdropfestival.tumblr.com/.

2018

AMOQA. Athens Museum of Queer Arts, Athens, Greece. https://amoqa.net/.
D21, Gallery, Leipzig, Germany. https://d21-leipzig.de/archive/index.php/ausstellungen--/225.html.

2020

Latvian Centre for Contemporary Art. Riga, Latvia. https://lcca.lv/en/.
Museum of Contemporary Art. Skopje, North Macedonia. https://msu.mk/home/.

Quadriennale di Roma. Palazzo delle Esposizioni, Rome, Italy. https://www.palazzoesposizioni.it.

2021

Art as Connection/Aargauer Kunsthaus, Aarau, Switzerland. https://www.aargauerkunsthaus.ch/en/exhibitions/2021/659.

District* Berlin. http://www.district-berlin.com.

CHAPTER 3

Feeling Brown, Feeling Down: Latina Affect, the Performativity of Race, and the Depressive Position

José Esteban Muñoz

Depression has become one of the dominant affective positions addressed within the cultural field of contemporary global capitalism. However, such a blanket statement requires fine-tuning. While art and media that depict the affective contours of depression have certainly become more prevalent, it is nonetheless important to be attentive to the ways in which the current historical moment is able to mimetically render various depictions of the problem of depression that plagues the contemporary citizen subject with a crypto-universalist script. Certainly depression is gendered. Female depression and male depression resonate quite differently. While female depression is more squarely framed as a problem, the depression that plagues men is often described as a full-on condition, registering

Originally printed in *Signs*, Vol. 31, No. 3, New Feminist Theories of Visual Culture (Spring 2006), pp. 675–688.

J. E. Muñoz (Deceased) (✉)
New York, NY, USA

J. Hollenbach and R. A. McDonald (eds.), *Re/Imagining Depression*,
https://doi.org/10.1007/978-3-030-80554-8_3

beyond the sphere of the individual, linked to a sort of angst and longing that are often described as endemic to postmodernism. However, that statement also requires some amending insofar as such a distinction reproduces a default white subject. The topic of depression has not often been discussed in relation to the question of racial formations in critical theory. This essay dwells on a particular depiction of depression that most certainly speaks to the general moment but resists the pull of crypto-universalism. The art project at the center of this essay considers how depression itself is formed and organized around various historical and material contingencies that include race, gender, and sex.

The work of Nao Bustamante does not conform to our associations of art practices that emerged at the moment of identity politics, nor does it represent an avoidance of the various antagonisms within the social that define our recognition and belonging as racialized, gendered, and sexed subjects. Bustamante's work tells us a story about the problems of belonging in alterity. I contend that her oeuvre meditates on our particularities, both shared and divergent, particularities that are central to the choreography of self and other that organizes our reality.[1] This, as I will contend, is negotiated through a particular affective circuit. The version of depression I consider in this essay is marked by a depression that is not one. I am provisionally naming this affective site a feeling of brownness that transmits and is structured through a depressive stance, a kind of feeling down, thus my rhyming title, "Feeling Brown, Feeling Down."

Bustamante's video installation "Neopolitan" (2003) includes an eleven-minute-long loop tape. The tape shows the artist breaking out into seemingly spontaneous sobbing as she watches the end of a movie. As she cries, the viewer witnesses the somatic signs of depressive sadness: her eyes well up, her nose runs. The video is shown on a monitor that sits on an old-fashioned table, which sits on a sculpture block. The monitor is covered by a multicolored cozy that was crocheted by the artist. On top of the cozy sits a crocheted basket filled with crocheted flowers. Above the basket rests an artificial crow; the artificial bird wears a matching crocheted hat. A power plug, connected to the wall, is also snugly covered in a crocheted caddy. The movie being watched by the artist is Tomás Gutiérrez Alea's "Fresa y chocolate" (1993), a film set in the 1970s in Cuba and focused on a difficult and fragile friendship between a proper revolutionary subject and a gay bohemian. As the artist watches the film, it is lightly projected on her face, giving the sense that the glow of the screen she is watching is bouncing off her face. After the film is over, the artist rewinds it again and again, continuing to cry.

In this essay I will suggest that this installation can be read as an illustration of the depressive position and its connection to minoritarian aesthetic and political practice. Toward this end I will draw from certain aspects of Kleinian object-relations theory. Thus, I will address a very particular mode of depression, not depression in its more general or clinical sense. Describing the depressive position in relation to what I am calling "brown feeling" chronicles a certain ethics of the self that is utilized and deployed by people of color and other minoritarian subjects who don't feel quite right within the protocols of normative affect and comportment. While the work of Melanie Klein (1986) and her circle is not tailored to attend to the vicissitudes of racialization and ethnic particularity, I nonetheless find some of her formulations suggestive and helpful when trying to discuss what I'm calling "brown feelings."

The larger project of this essay engages different psychological and phenomenological discourses in an effort to theorize affective particularity and belonging. Jonathan Flatley (2004) has recently described his own interest in affective particularity in relation to the social as affective mapping. Affective mapping is Flatley's amplification and amendment of Fredric Jameson's (1981) theory of cognitive mapping. To some degree such a description would hold sway with this analysis. My endeavor, more descriptively, is intended to enable a project that imagines a position or narrative of being and becoming that can resist the pull of identitarian models of relationality. Affect is not meant to be a simple placeholder for identity in my work. Indeed, it is supposed to be something altogether different; it is, instead, supposed to be descriptive of the receptors we use to hear each other and the frequencies on which certain subalterns speak and are heard or, more importantly, felt. This leaves us to amend Gayatri Chakravorty Spivak's famous question, "Can the subaltern speak?" (1988, 1999) to ask How does the subaltern feel? How might subalterns feel each other? Toward this end, modified theories of object relations can potentially translate into productive ways in which to consider relationality within a larger social sphere.

Certain acts of translation must happen if we are to use Klein to consider feeling brown or any other modality of minoritarian being or becoming. This entails addressing what I have mentioned as the crypto-universal aspect of various aesthetic and hermeneutical projects. A touchstone for this aspect of my work is the writing of Hortense Spillers.

In her powerful meditation on psychoanalysis and race, "All the Things You Could Be by Now if Sigmund Freud's Wife Was Your Mother," the literary theorist deuniversalizes psychoanalytic tools in generative ways:

> Is it not, then, the task of a psychoanalytical protocol to effect a translation from the muteness of desire/wish—that which shames and baffles the subject, even if its origins are dim, not especially known—into an articulated syntactic particularity? This seems to me a passable psychoanalytic goal, but perhaps there is more to it than simply a nice thing to happen? At the very least I am suggesting that an aspect of the emancipatory project hinges on what would appear to be a simple self-attention, except that reaching the articulation requires a process, that of making one's subjectness the object of a disciplined and potentially displaceable attentiveness. (2003, p. 400).

Her understatement here is poignant—it would indeed be much more than "simply a nice thing" for groups and circuits of belonging to leave the realm of muteness and attain a valuable "articulated syntactic particularity" that is tuned to group identification. Thus for Spillers, the psychoanalytical protocol is laden with an emancipatory potentiality in that it helps one combat a certain muteness that social logics like homophobia, racism, and sexism would project onto the minoritarian subject. This move to identify the radical impulse in developmental theories aims to recast the theories outside the parameters of positivism and enact their political performativity for circuits of belonging that do not conform to a crypto-universalism associated with the universal white subject. Spillers's argument confirms that a hermeneutical approach that is indeed attentive to psychoanalytic questions may provide descriptions of our own recognition via the route of racial performativity. Racial performativity is the final key concept that this essay foregrounds. The meaning I am assigning to the term racial performativity is intended to get at an aspect of race that is "a doing."[2] More precisely, I mean to describe a political doing, the effects that the recognition of racial belonging, coherence, and divergence present in the world. This turn to the performativity of race has to do with the fact that during this moment where the discourse of race is prone to the corrosive forces of corporate multiculturalism and other manifestations of globalization, it seems especially important to consider racial formations through a lens that is not hamstrung by positivism, insofar as the discourse of positivism is at best reductive and unresponsive to the particularities of racial formations. The epistemological core of what race is has become less and less accessible during these tumultuous times. It is therefore expedient to consider what race does. Furthermore, to look at race as a performative enterprise, one that can best be accessed by its effects, may lead us out of political and conceptual impasses that have dogged racial discourse. A critical project attuned to knowing the performativity of race is indeed better suited to decipher what work race does in the world.

What I am describing as "feeling brown, feeling down" is a modality of recognizing the racial performativity generated by an affective particularity that is coded to specific historical subjects who can provisionally be recognized by the term *Latina*. Feeling brown in my analysis is descriptive of the ways in which minoritarian affect is always, no matter what its register, partially illegible in relation to the normative affect performed by normative citizen subjects. The notion of brownness has been rendered differently by essayist Richard Rodriguez, who is also interested in describing brownness in relation to a certain antinormativity. In his most recent (2003) book, the Mexican American memoirist revisits the scene of his racialized upbringing in California and his feelings of nonbelonging to a majoritarian sphere. His narrative uses race (and to a much lesser degree queerness) as a springboard to discuss the particularity of being brown. Yet he leaps so far away from a racially situated notion of this affective phenomenon that brownness becomes the justification for Rodriguez's identification with Richard Nixon over John F. Kennedy during their famous televised debate of 1960. My approach to brownness does not correspond with Rodriguez's work on this ideological level. More nearly, thinking through brownness is akin to what Spillers describes as the "making of one's subjectness the object of a disciplined and potentially displaceable attentiveness" (2003, p. 400). Brown feelings are not individualized affective particularity; they more nearly express this "displaceable attentiveness," which is to say a larger collective mapping of self and other. Aesthetic practices enable these mapping protocols. In my current research project, I am interested in all sorts of antinormative feelings that correspond to minoritarian becoming. In some cases aesthetic practices and performances offer a particular theoretical lens to understand the ways in which different circuits of belonging connect, which is to say that recognition flickers between minoritarian subjects. Brownness is not white, and it is not black either, yet it does not simply sit midway between them. Brownness, like all forms of racialized attentiveness in North America, is enabled by practices of self-knowing formatted by the nation's imaginary through the powerful spikes in the North American consciousness identified with the public life of blackness. At the same time, brownness is a mode of attentiveness to the self for others that is cognizant of the way in which it is not and can never be whiteness. Whiteness in my analysis is also very specific: I read it as a cultural logic that prescribes and regulates national feelings and comportment. White is thus an affective gauge that helps us understand some modes of emotional countenance and comportment as good or bad. It should go without saying that some modes of whiteness—for example, working-class whiteness—are stigmatized within the majoritarian public sphere. Modes of white womanhood or white ethnicities do not correspond with the affective ruler that measures and naturalizes white feelings as the norm.

Depression is not brown, but there are modalities of depression that seem quite brown. Psychoanalytic critic Antonio Viego (2003) has looked at how American ego psychology attempts to perform a certain kind of therapeutic work on Latino/a subjects. The telos of that project is to achieve a gradually realized whole and well-adjusted minority self. The majority of ego-psychological work explored by Viego attempts to translate notions of traditional Latino maladies—*los nervios and attaques*—into ethnically named translations of disorders analyzed as depression and anxiety disorder in English and North American institutional formats. Viego's critique dismantles this wish for an ego that is not shattered in Latino psychology. For Viego, such a desire would be an escape from the social. Thus, any social theory that posits happiness as its goal is a flawed theory. Viego's use of psychoanalytic protocols functions as a displaceable attentiveness that imagines a mode of brown politics not invested in the narrative of a whole and well-adjusted subject.

My notion of feeling down is meant to be a translation of the idea of a depressive position. Thus, down is a way to link position with feeling. The use of the concept of positions, rather than the more developmental discourses on stages, is one of Klein's (1986) amendments to Freud. Scholars interested in Klein or object-relations psychology view positions, as opposed to stages, as less turgid trajectories of emotional development. In this instance Klein's contribution resonates alongside one of Antonio Gramsci's most substantial contributions to social theory, namely, his thinking about the war of positions as a mode of resistance that is different from the classical Marxian revolt described as a war of maneuvers (1996 [1992]). Positions in both theorists' lexicons are provisional and flexible demarcations, practices of being.

The depressive position for Klein is not a stage that must be moved beyond. There are ways in which such occupations of the depressive position lead to reparation, where love helps one surpass paranoid and schizoid feelings. In infancy the child splits the maternal other into two objects. One is a good breast that represents a continuous flow of fulfillment—a sense of being one with the mother. Yet the fact that such a flow is not continuous leads to feelings of resentment and hate toward what becomes the bad breast. For Klein these destructive feelings vector into a sort of cannibalistic or sadistic urge. The infant later feels considerable guilt about possessing such destructive feelings. At some point the split object becomes, once again, whole, and the child is able to once again introject it. The object, like the subject, is never whole, but the fiction or feeling of wholeness is crucial for survival within the social. In her 1946 paper "Notes on Some Schizoid Mechanisms" Klein explains that "the drive to make reparation, which comes to the fore at this stage, can be regarded as a consequence of a greater insight into psychic reality and of growing synthesis, for it shows a more realistic response to feelings of grief, guilt and fear of loss resulting from the loved object. Since the drive to repair or protect the injured object paves the way for more satisfactory object relations and sublimations, it in turn increases synthesis between inner and external situations" (1986 [1946], p. 189).

The depressive position is, in Kleinian theory, associated with a kind of interjection, which is a stark opposite to the practice of projecting menace or threat as exterior to the self. The depressive position is not a linear or task-oriented sense of developmental closure. It is instead a position that we live in, and it describes the ways in which we attempt to enter psychic reality, where we can see objects as whole, both interior and exterior, not simply as something that hums outside our existence. To extend, or in Spillers's phraseology, "displace," this attentiveness of the self to others is to begin to understand one of the deep functions of brown feelings, to see the other in alterity as existing in a relational field to the self. In this sense I am proposing an ethics of brownness, one that attempts to incorporate understandings of the psychic in the service of understanding the social. The whole object that is interjected in the depressive position is not real, or more nearly, not firmly bound. One always feels its drive toward fragmentation, but taking up the depressive position is one way in which, as subjects, we resist a disrepair within the social that would lead to a breakdown in one's ability to see and know the other. That would certainly be a mode of clinical depression.

In queer studies Eve Kosofsky Sedgwick (2003) has recently turned to the divide between paranoia and reparation. Sedgwick has argued that paranoia has become a standardized posture taken in queer critique and that it thus has become routine rather than critical thinking. The paranoid move is always about a certain hermeneutic unveiling of an external threat. Such a move becomes routine, or numb repetition, and renders the paranoid subject unable to participate in what Spillers would call the intra-mural protocol of a displaceable self-attentiveness. Spillers (2003) wishes to turn away from a critique of "the man" and turn to a theory of the way in which relational skills are organized around "the one." The one, for Spillers, is interior to the life world of the black community, the lives we have among one another within racial formations. This is not to say that there are not multiple threats presented by an outsider, by the man, but Spillers want us to understand the ways in which our own sense of relationality and practices of belonging within communities of color are threatened from within. Spillers in this instance is once again insisting on repealing a certain paranoid sense of being in the world where menace is exterior to our world of intraracial or ethnic experience and instead wants to linger or dwell in the realm of this enabling fantasy of a whole object.

Sedgwick invites her readers and the field of queer critique to consider reparation. In this same intervention Sedgwick wishes to consider how certain strong theories of the social, theories that can be codified as prescriptive and totalizing, might not be as advantageous at this particular moment as weak theories that do not position themselves in the same masterful, totalizing fashion. I would align a Gramscian war of positions with this weak theory. I understand the theory-making impulse that propels my description of feeling brown as resisting the strong-theory model. The stitching I am doing between critical race theories, queer critique, and psychological object-relations theory is a provisional and heuristic approach that wishes to stave off the totalizing aspect of all those modes of critique.

I want to suggest that the ethics of "the one" that Spillers rehearses is a mode of intramural depressive positionality that gives us the ability to know and experience the other who shares a particular affective or emotional valence with us. The reparation staged in Spillers's theoretical work is informed by a desire to return to another place that she describes as "old-fashioned." *Old-fashioned* is associated with the nonsecular belonging that in turn is associated with the history of the black church (2003). Spillers explicitly desires a secular space where such relationality is possible, but *old-fashioned* is not only deployed in its conventional usage, it is also written in a psychic sense—the desire for a moment before communities of color lapsed into functional impasse. This functional impasse is certainly relational to a well-founded sense of paranoia and also to the ways in which such continuous challenges within the social spur a disconnect from psychic reality where our relational potentiality is diminished. This turn to the old-fashioned in Spillers, this desire for "the one," is a desire that is relational to a depressive position that does not succumb to a paranoid-schizoid position. The depressive position in Klein is the ethical position. Taking that point into account, I would argue that feeling brown, feeling down is an ethical position within the social for the minoritarian subject.

My stitching together of theories, my attempt at weaving together a provisional whole that is indeed not a whole but rather an enabling sense of wholeness that allows a certain level of social recognition, is a reparative performance. However, one should be cognizant of the three different modes of reparation that Klein distinguishes. It is useful to break these types down. One is a kind of manic reparation that carries a sense of triumph, since it essentially flips over the child-parent relationship at the parent's expense. Another notion of the reparative is a mode of obsessive reparation that can be characterized as compulsive repetition, a sort of placating magical thinking. Finally, there is the type of reparation that I wish to promote for the fields of inquiry discussed in this essay. This modality is what I see at work in Bustamante's installation. This would be a form of reparation that is grounded in love for the object. Klein argues that "one moment after we have seen the most sadistic impulses, we meet with performances showing the greatest capacity for love and the wish to make all possible sacrifices to be loved" (1986 [1935], p. 124). Utilizing Klein as a theorist of relationality is advantageous because she is true to the facts of violence, division, and hierarchy that punctuate the social, yet she is, at another moment, a deeply idealistic thinker who understands the need to not simply cleanse negativity but instead to promote the desire that the subject has in the wake of the negative to reconstruct a relational field. Love for Klein is thus not just a romantic abstraction; it is indeed a kind of striving for belonging that does not ignore the various obstacles that the subject must overcome to achieve the most provisional belonging.

"Neopolitan," Bustamante's installation, is stitched together by a homey crocheted binding that seems elastic and permeable, its texture reminiscent of a nostalgia for a mode of domesticity associated with hobbyism, with craft and domestic forms of belonging. The texture of the installation is meant to connote a sense of home and belonging that is perhaps squarely in the past, yet it nonetheless wishes to recirculate that sense of belonging in relation to our presentness and our futurity. While not a cynical assemblage, the object is not without a sense of humor. The sad crow of depression, a species that is quite apart from the bluebird of happiness, wears a snug little bonnet that links him to the odd object over which he sits watch. It is a construct as elaborate and provisional as the selves we perform within the social. The fact that a monitor is enshrouded by a homemade covering indexes the ways in which televisual reality is linked to real life and fantasy. The homey fabric enfolding the television set indicates that home is where the heart is, and at the center of this home we will find a television set.

The video on the loop and the performance of sobbing, rewinding, and sobbing again is a performance of repetition. Repetition is the piece's most obvious depressive quality. It describes the ways in which subjects occupy and dwell within the depressive position. The piece's play of light, the illumination bathing the artist's face, and the illumination that the object itself offers comment on a complicated choreography of interjection and projection. The sound track that washes over the artist and, in turn, the viewer is the familiar swelling associated with melodrama, the weepy, the woman's film, and this track, in relation to this installation, is the sound of brown feelings.

The film being screened in the video, the source of the sadness and somatic excess, is a Cuban film about homosexuality and revolution. Its tragedy has to do with the way in which queerness can finally not be held by the nation-state. This is the rip, the moment of breakdown in a revolutionary imaginary. In a similar fashion, this is a rip or break in the object-relation theories that I have been considering. In the bulk of this work, in Klein, D. W. Winnicott, and others who came after Freud, homosexuality is a primitive condition that needs to be contained, managed, or surpassed. Queerness is the site of emotional breakdown and the activation of the melodrama in the installation. I would thus position Bustamante's art object as a corrective in relation to the homophobic developmental plot. Queerness, the installation shows, never fully disappears; instead, it haunts the present. More nearly, it is something whose mourning is a condition of possibility for other modes of sexuality that are less problematic.

All of this mourning comes out of a specific time and place, which is to say that it is historically situated. To illustrate this point, I turn to a moment in London, during a question-and-answer session following an artist's talk in which Bustamante discussed "Neopolitan." When the artist fielded the question "How is your work different from that of Bas Jan Ader, another artist who represented his tears?" I wanted to answer the question for the artist, but, fulfilling my role as critic and onlooker, I could not. I nonetheless take this opportunity to do so in hope of explaining not only the difference between two art projects, spread apart by thirty years, but also to remark on the value of displaceable attentiveness in relation to aesthetics and psychoanalysis. Ader mysteriously disappeared at sea in 1975 as part of his performance project. Depression, sadness, and loss saturate his work. The three-minute black-and-white film "I Am Too Sad to Tell You" (1971) is reminiscent of Bustamante's crying tape. It portrays the artist driven to tears and crying for a prolonged time. The motivation behind his emotion is left even more ambiguous than the themes that constitute Bustamante's installation. Ader's performance rehearses something that is very much like the ethics of Klein's depressive position. Ader's work is beautiful and moving. It seduces us with the lure of the universal. These tears are not wrapped up in the kind of affective particularity that I associate with brownness and queerness in my reading of "Neopolitan." I reference "I Am Too Sad to Tell You" in an effort to illustrate the ways in which some tears access a universal sadness or loss that offers us a generalized story of the world of affect, stopping short of linking affect to historical loss. What motivates these tears? Loss and history become untethered in Ader's film. While "Neopolitan" certainly speaks across particularities within the social, it addresses a historical particularity, one that I describe as a feeling, feeling down.

Jennifer Doyle (2005) skillfully compares Ader's work with that of feminist artist Marina Abramovic's video performance "The Onion" (1995) and Hayley Newman's "Crying Glasses (An Aid to Melancholia)" (1995). In Abramovic's piece the lauded performance artist lists complaints about her life, ones that are not very interesting, banalities like time spent in waiting rooms and the annoyances that accompany travel. Newman's performance is one of her artificial performances, fake performances that are documented as if they were real in a series she calls Connotations Performance. However, the distinction between the two women artists' works and Ader's, as described by Doyle, is instructive when thinking through the historicizing of affect and tears:

> As the title reminds us (telling us that the artist won't tell us), we do not know why Ader is crying. As a male artist with a particular mythology (he disappeared while attempting to sail across the Atlantic in execution of a performance), Bas Jan Ader is closer to the eighteenth-century ideal of the gentlemanly "man of feeling" than he is to the female melodrama cited by Abramovic. The portrait is an extension of his interest in the subject of his own vulnerability (as in a series of short films that document the artist falling over—riding a bicycle into a canal, falling from a tree, standing and swaying from side to side until he falls down). His film, when compared with Newman's photograph or Abramovic's performance, comes off as more purely seductive—and as somehow more private—in part because nothing in the film indicates that we must read it as "produced" for the camera. (2005, pp. 48–49)

The man of feeling is a universal subject. The spectator cannot know what his tears are about because they are deeply private, as Doyle indicates, as is the very nature of the tear. However, they are also universal tears in the ways in which Newman's are false tears (the tears of feminine deception) or Abramovic's are onion-peeling kitchen tears (the tears that mark women's work). Doyle, citing Jameson (1981), reminds readers that "history is what hurts" (Doyle 2005, p. 50). We are then left to contemplate which histories are marked by particular tears and which histories are elided. In the remainder of this essay, I will discuss an attempt to get at the performativity of brownness that marks Bustamante's tears.

In a review for *Artweek*, Lindsay Westbrook discusses the installation in terms that help make visible what outside contingencies get projected onto Bustamante's piece by its audience:

> Nao Bustamante's 'Neopolitan' is also brand new and deals with several themes that recur in her work; emotionality, vulnerability and stereotypes of gender and Mexican-American culture; we watch her watching a scene from the Cuban film 'Strawberries and Chocolate.' She is making herself cry, periodically rewinding the tape and wiping her eyes on a Mexican flag hanky. The work is profoundly self-conscious, of course, and, for that reason, cynical. But it is also genuinely sad, expressing sorrow and mourning, perhaps, for the current world situation. (2003, p. 14)

The dynamics of projection in this thumbnail sketch are worth looking at for a couple of reasons. The hanky that the reviewer identifies as the Mexican flag is no such thing. It is merely a colored dish towel. The fact that Bustamante's Mexicanness was projected onto her installation does in fact make a case for the various ways in which brown paranoia is not something that can be wished away, no matter how much we would like to fully escape the regime of paranoia. Indeed, the brown depressive position I'm describing is called into being in relation to the various projections screened on the embodied self from the outside. The formulation, in which self-consciousness equals cynicism, is odd. Yet the lines with which Westbrook closes her analysis do bear remembering. Indeed this mode of sadness has a great deal to do with the "world situation." That is, the video represents and performs a political depression, which is neither a clinical depression nor a literal breakdown. This political recognition contains a reparative impulse that I want to describe as enabling and liberatory, in the same way that an attentiveness to those things mute within us, brought into language and given a syntax, can potentially lead to an insistence on change and political transformation.

In discussing the depressive position, Julia Kristeva (2004) reminds Klein's readers that reparation is far from idyllic, since the purportedly whole object is tainted with despair. The object's state of disintegration is never fully resolved. It is instead worked through. Certainly "Neopolitan" is nothing like an ideal aesthetic object, but it does represent a creative impulse, where grief is temporally conjoined to ideas. In this essay I've attempted to suggest the various ways in which the depressive position is a site of potentiality and not simply a breakdown of the self or the social fabric. Reparation is part of the depressive position; it signals a certain kind of hope. The depressive position is a tolerance of the loss and guilt that underlies the subject's sense of self—which is to say that it does not avoid or wish away loss and guilt. It is a position in which the subject negotiates reality, resisting the instinct to fall into the delusional realm of the paranoid schizoid. I have also attempted to call attention to the ways in which minoritarian chains of recognition can benefit from avoiding paranoid positions that keep them from engaging the necessary project of being attentive to the self in an effort to know the other, but indeed my central goal has been one of enacting and performing a sort of reparative analysis that describes and bolsters the project of feeling brown. The depressive position, as described in the work of Klein and adjusted through Spillers's questions, offers a useful insight into one dimension of what I am calling feeling brown. Feeling brown is a mode of racial performativity, a doing within the social that surpasses limitations of epistemological renderings of race.

Notes

1. This word usage is calibrated to address a minoritarian subject. For more on this particular narrative of subjectivity, see Muñoz (1999).
2. This idea of performativity as "a doing" is indebted to a line of thought in the post-disciplinary field of performance studies that engages the work of the philosopher of everyday speech, J. L. Austin, and his book *How to Do Things with Words* (1962). See Parker and Sedgwick (1995) for a useful introduction to some of Austin's postdisciplinary relevance.

References

Abramovic, Marina. 1995. *The Onion*. Video art. Independently produced.

Ader, Bas Jan, director. 1971. *I Am Too Sad to Tell You*. 16 mm black-and-white film, silent; 3 minutes 21 seconds. Independently produced.

Austin, J.L. 1962. *How to Do Things with Words*. Oxford: Clarendon.

Bustamante, Nao. 2003. *Neopolitan*. Performance art. Independently produced.

Doyle, Jennifer. 2005. Critical Tears: Melodrama and Museums. In *Getting Emotional*, ed. Nicholas Baume, 42–53. Boston: Institute of Contemporary Art.

Flatley, Jonathan. 2004. Reading into Henry James. *Criticism* 46 (1): 103–123.

Gramsci, Antonio. 1996 [1992]. *The Prison Notebooks*, ed. Joseph A. Buttigieg and trans. Joseph A. Buttigieg and Antonio Callari. New York: Columbia University Press.

Jameson, Fredric. 1981. *The Political Unconscious: Narrative as a Socially Symbolic Act*. Ithaca, NY: Cornell University Press.

Klein, Melanie. 1986 [1935]. The Psychogenesis of Manic-Depressive States. In *Klein 1986*, 115–145.

———. 1986 [1946]. Notes on Schizoid Mechanisms. In *Klein 1986*, 175–200.

———. 1986. *The Selected Melanie Klein*, ed. Juliet Mitchell. New York: Free Press.

Kristeva, Julia. 2004. *Melanie Klein*, trans. Ross Guberman. New York: Columbia University Press.

Muñoz, José Esteban. 1999. *Disidentifications: Queers of Color and the Performance of Politics*. Minneapolis: University of Minnesota Press.

Newman, Hayley. 1995. *Crying Glasses (An Aid to Melancholia)*. Performance art. From the series *Connotations* Performance. Screened at the Ikon Gallery, Birmingham, UK.

Parker, Andrew, and Eve Kosofsky Sedgwick. 1995. Introduction: Performativity and Performance. In *Performativity and Performance*, 1–18. New York: Routledge.

Rodriguez, Richard. 2003. *Brown: The Last Discovery of America*. New York: Penguin.
Sedgwick, Eve Kosofsky. 2003. *Touching Feeling: Affect, Pedagogy, Performativity*. Durham, NC: Duke University Press.
Spillers, Hortense. 2003. "All the Things You Could Be by Now If Sigmund Freud's Wife Was Your Mother": Psychoanalysis and Race. In *Black, White, and in Color: Essays on American Literature and Culture*, 376–428. Chicago: University of Chicago Press.
Spivak, Gayatri Chakravorty. 1988. "Can the Subaltern Speak?" In *Marxism and the Interpretation of Culture*, ed. Cary Nelson and Lawrence Grossberg, 271–313. Chicago: University of Chicago Press.
———. 1999. *A Critique of Postcolonial Reason*. Cambridge, MA: Harvard University Press.
Viego, Antonio. 2003. The Unconscious of Latino/a Studies. *Latino Studies* 1 (3): 333–336.
Westbrook, Lindsay. 2003. Review. *Artweek* 34 (10): 14.

CHAPTER 4

Not Down but Different: Depression in the Shadow of the Black Dog

John Streamas

Our small table scarcely accommodated the three of us already gathered for lunch when Janet arrived (Janet is a pseudonym). She was catching her breath as she sat and asked whether we had heard the news about Iris Chang. This was November 2004, and we were in Atlanta for the annual conference of the American Studies Association. On separate panels Janet and I had presented papers on Japanese Americans' wartime incarceration; and all of us at the table knew Iris Chang's books on Chinese Americans and wartime Japanese atrocities in China. Janet told us that Chang had committed suicide. Through lunch we sat stunned and quiet. None of us had known Chang or had even seen her at a reading or presentation. Yet we felt a connection to her, defined not so much by race—three of us are Asian American, but Janet is white—as by our admiration for a passion that distinguished the scholarship of her controversial 1997 book *The Rape of Nanking*. (As recently as November 2017, Randy Hopkins issued

J. Streamas (✉)
School of Languages, Cultures, and Race, Washington State University, Pullman, WA, USA
e-mail: streamas@wsu.edu

J. Hollenbach and R. A. McDonald (eds.), *Re/Imagining Depression*,
https://doi.org/10.1007/978-3-030-80554-8_4

a lengthy essay accusing many U.S. historians of yielding to Japanese government propaganda's claims of Chang's "errors and poor quality" [p. 1].)

Such connections seem rare in academia. As graduate students we are drawn to fields to which, because they engage us, we devote our working lives, yet we are also taught that the best, most responsible scholarship is dispassionate and disinterested, fair and reliable because it is objective. To evolve our devotion to a field into a personal investment, a position on a controversial issue, is implicitly unethical, no less than a football coach's acceptance of a sponsorship from a shoe company that exploits sweatshop labor or a microbiologist's acceptance of research funding from a pharmaceutical company that charges consumers impossible prices for life-saving treatments. The difference is that coaches and scientists who engage in such practices are usually rewarded by their gratefully oblivious institutions, while an African American professor of Ethnic Studies is reprimanded for protesting institutional policy that defends the hate speech of campus bigots. The difference is that when the professor is targeted for racial harassment and even threats by right-wing groups, the university refuses to defend her. Instead, she is told that taking a controversial political position is antithetical to good scholarship and that the university is not obligated to protect her. For this reason, even in fields such as Ethnic Studies and History, few scholars take stands as passionate as Iris Chang's, and of those who do, most work on the fringes of academia, or even outside it, as independent scholars. The few of us who try to exercise our commitments from within "the belly of the beast" know that there is no safety net even in our own departments. We know that there are risks involved, and that one of those risks is depression.

* * *

Much has been made of the current "age of Trump" in the United States and the world. Racism and xenophobia, though never exactly well hidden, have risen boldly to the surface of cultural and political life. And despite the far right's attacks on higher education, university administrators usually try to accommodate and even placate conservative political leaders. To sustain their customer base of students, they fortify their provision of mental health services, which they require faculty to advertise; however, they do little to improve such services to faculty themselves. In this time of extreme cultural and political tension on college campuses, some scholars are investigating the mental health of faculty. Margaret Price and Stephanie L. Kerschbaum devote a report to "faculty with mental illnesses," and their purpose is to recommend ways of improving "campus climate" that are "directed primarily toward *environments* and *attitudes* rather than toward individual people" (original emphasis, 2017, p. 5). Those recommendations stress access and inclusiveness. Given the research-oriented setting of academic work, they report, distressingly but unsurprisingly, that studies of faculty suffering mental illness are rare, but they suggest that rates of attrition and unemployment "are likely to be high" (Price and Kerschbaum 2017, p. 7).

Price and Kerschbaum discuss mental illnesses generally rather than depression in particular, though it can be surmised that even as the most prevalent of mental illnesses, depression among faculty is still understudied. Similarly, as a scholar of race and ethnicity, I know that campus diversity policies as they affect faculty of color have only recently begun to receive rigorous scrutiny. Given these two understudied areas, I argue that depression among faculty of color is similarly neglected. Teaching Ethnic Studies, I know that many students of color who might benefit from mental health services refuse to seek help because they do not trust institutions, even when those institutions claim to offer culture-specific help. We have all grown distrustful of diversity programs and policies that make big promises and fail to deliver. In my own university, a new president vowed to improve campus climate by acceding to student protestors' demand that many more faculty of color be hired—the third of four goals toward "diversity and inclusion" listed by the president in September 2017 is to "implement a hiring plan to increase the number of faculty and staff of color"—but in a message delivering budget news in October 2017 the president mandated cuts of "2.5 percent" in each unit, which indicates that the number of faculty of color is likelier to decrease rather than increase (Schulz 29 September; Schulz 23 October). While students of color comprise between one-fourth and one-third of all students on this rural southeast Washington campus, faculty of color comprise, by the president's own acknowledgement, less than ten percent of all faculty. The wonder, then, is not why so few people of color access institutional services such as those that support mental health, but why any do at all.

The American Psychological Association finds that "Asian Americans are less likely to seek help for their emotional or mental health problems than whites," and being Japanese American myself, this research speaks to my own experiences and findings (Meyers 2006, p. 44). Research into causes of mental health issues in Asian Americans is only preliminary, and explanations are therefore vague and broad. Psychologists hesitate to advance analyses. But the artists, activists, and scholars who contribute to a recent issue of *Asian American Literary Review* hold back nothing. Kai Cheng Thom writes, "Mental health is the language of power—the power to exist within, and sometimes define, the conventions of sanity, normalcy, the status quo, capitalism, white heteropatriarchy" (2016, p. 9). The biology of illness is real, Thom argues, but sources of mental illness "greater than biological illness or personal failure" are sure to be found in "colonization, capitalism, racial and gendered violence" (2016, p. 11). In an essay titled "Diversity Work," Cynthia Wu, who identifies as Asian and genderqueer, writes about students at her university protesting a hostile racial climate. Although administrators agreed to form a committee that would meet with the protestors, which Wu joined, she left it at year's end because "[n]othing has changed to make the university more hospitable for students of color. We're just covering the dirt on the floor—not rebuilding from the ground up" (2016, p. 42). As a tenured scholar, Wu notes that, "Diversity work in universities asks us to hide—not solve—problems," and she challenges fellow scholars of color with troubling questions: "At what cost to us do we keep cleaning up—the listening, the empathizing, the offering of the tissue box—when colleges and universities fail? At what cost to us do we acquiesce to complicity with the sweep under the rug that these institutions expect" (2016, p. 42).

Thom speaks openly of a suicide attempt, as do others writing in *Asian American Literary Review*. The stereotype of the "model minority"—the idea that Asian Americans prosper because of their superior work ethic and uncomplaining spirit—bears the downside of young Asians struggling with parental pressure to be the best. The stereotype individuates Asian Americans against cultural expectations, refusing to see that they inhabit a world governed by the "colonization, capitalism, racial and gendered violence" that Thom diagnoses and the institutional indifference that Wu condemns. Stereotypes cannot account for the fact that in the United States, "[a]mong females 15–24 years old, Asian Americans and Pacific Islanders (AAPIs) have the highest rate of suicide deaths (14.1%) compared to other racial/ethnic groups"—considerably higher than women categorized as Black and Hispanic—and that "AAPI males in the same age range have the second highest rate of suicide deaths" (Lee et al. 2009, p. 145). Cultural stereotypes suggest that Asian Americans regard institutional help as somehow disgraceful, a sign of personal failing, but surely the reason that many Asian Americans do not report their depression is no different from their reason for failing to report episodes of racial harassment: they distrust the system. I can cite no corroborating studies, but I suspect that Asian Americans seek institutional help only as a desperate last resort—as Iris Chang did.

Chang's white friend and admirer Paula Kamen devoted a book, *Finding Iris Chang*, to wondering why Chang killed herself. In the end, Kamen attributes Chang's death to a predictable multiplicity of causes but suggests that the illness of bipolar disorder "was probably the main villain behind Iris' death" (2007, p. 271). This is the very sort of diagnosis that Kai Cheng Thom might dismiss, but then even Kamen concedes, "desperately lacking is research and public awareness about how gender and ethnicity can shape mood disorders" (p. 272).

Immigrant Chinese American fiction writer Yiyun Li published her first book-length nonfiction in the form of a depression memoir. In my research it was, until very recently, one of only two depression memoirs by an Asian American author, and one of very few such books by an American writer of color. By "depression memoir" I mean the genre of personal narratives of depression. Obviously, all writers of color who consider race and racism are writing about a major source of depression. All through the works of writers such as Morrison and Baldwin are causes of depression. But these works do not fit under the category "depression memoir" as do books such as Styron's *Darkness Visible* (1989), Solomon's *The Noonday Demon* (2015), Merkin's *This Close to Happy* (2017), and many others by middle-class whites. (Another, recent depression memoir by an Asian American woman, written as personal essays, is Esmé Weijun Wang's *The Collected Schizophrenias* [2019]. Still another by a writer of color is the immigrant Meri Nana-Ama Danquah's *Willow Weep for Me: A Black Woman's Journey Through Depression* [1998].)

Li's work is ostensibly a record of her two hospitalizations for suicidal depression. Her self-description offers insight not only into the anti-individualist aspect of Chinese culture but also into possible effects on a Chinese American woman novelist: "A word I hate to use in English is *I*. It is a melodramatic word. In Chinese, a language less grammatically strict, one can construct a sentence with an implied subject pronoun and skip that embarrassing *I*, or else replace it with *we*. Living is not an original business" (original emphasis, 2017, p. 27). This last sentence seems not to belong to the three sentences preceding it, and yet it modifies those sentences so that they lose their quality of self-effacement. They instead become a striving for identification. Two paragraphs later Li writes that "for months after the hospital stays I tried to explain to those around me that anyone can be, and should be, replaceable" (p. 27). To identify with everyone, dead and living, can involve a replaceability that is affirmative, not self-erasing. And yet Li is also immersed sufficiently in Western culture so that, bridging cultures, she understands the gravity of disappearance: "time spent with other people is the time to prepare for their disappearance. That there is an opposite perspective I can only understand theoretically. The timeline is also a repetition of one's lapse into isolation. It's not others who vanish, but from others one vanishes" (p. 36). This is the sort of racial and cultural difference that, as a cause of depression, is most likely overlooked in the Western psychological literature.

The relationship between others and the Asian self that troubles Li points to a serious problem in the "model minority" stereotype. When the Asian exceeds the white standard, there are only other high-achieving Asians to compete with. Not all can be the best, and so most fall into the trap of "Asianfail," a term I first encountered in the title of Eleanor Ty's study of narratives of Asian American "failure" in literature and film. I encountered it again in Urban Dictionary, where the first definition is, "To not get an A in a class." On her first page Ty demonstrates that, on social media, the term names Asian Americans' "insider jokes about their own inability to pick up food with chopsticks, to cook rice, or to shine at math and computers" (2017, p. 1). But Ty also sees these "as ambivalent articulations of contemporary Asian North American youthful subjectivity—not of a sense of a mortifying failure to belong, but of a vacillation between embarrassment and pride in not conforming to or belonging to anything imagined as 'Asian.' They reveal a sense of relief in their failure to comply with normative expectations of being Asian" (p. 23). The "vacillation between embarrassment and pride" confines Asian Americans to being neither wholly Asian nor wholly American—neither the model nor the standard, and I suspect that "vacillation" is often accompanied by depression, and for some, by attempts at suicide. Indeed, Andrew Solomon quietly observes that "East Asians ... avoid the subject [of depression] to the point of abject denial" (2015, p. 200).

* * *

"The black dog" is a now-common metaphor of depression, but an online search discovers several early applicants of it: Samuel Johnson,

English folklore, Roman poets, Greek and Egyptian and Middle Eastern mythologies (for an accessible example, see "The History of the 'Black Dog' as Metaphor" in Joshua Preston's *A Prairie Populist* Website [2013]). The "black dog syndrome" names a narrative by which, in animal shelters, black dogs are last to be adopted and most commonly euthanized; and, though the narrative has been credibly countered by advocates who charge it with statistical inadequacy, I still find it significant that a writer for *Slate*, Katy Waldman, calls the syndrome a kind of racism (2014).

In Ethnic Studies I examine links between discourses of color and of race. Asians, for example, have been colored yellow in the minds of European colonizers (Keevak 2011). I have been struck by the fact that, among the four ancient bodily fluids, the biles are black and yellow. Melancholy was linked to "an excess of black bile" (Solomon 2015, p. 286). Though black has not always been linked to death and decay and evil, the linkage is still so common that even Andrew Solomon, in his memoir and history of depression, refers to what he calls Samuel Johnson's "blackest depressions" (p. 310).

Herein lies a great irony of the discourse of mental illness: that, while research into the relationship between race and depression is sparse, and while depression memoirs remain a genre practiced mostly by white middle-class writers, a metaphor common in the discourse of illness shares many negative definitions with a figure common in the discourse of race. "African Americans in the seventies," writes Anne Anlin Cheng, "were encouraged to internalize the Black Is Beautiful credo and to fight actively against discrimination rather than to permit the degradation of the self" (2001, p. 5). And yet, immobilized by depression, some African Americans were still chased by "the black dog."

Is black a presence or an absence of all colors? It has traditionally been regarded as a color of death, but then death is also called a shadow, a force in shades, and shadows have no inherent colors. This may be the point, though: that just as death has no real color, so too does a condition of suicidal despair have no real color. One condition of marginalization is invisibility, identified most famously in the title of Ralph Ellison's novel *Invisible Man* (1952)—and invisibility is also an absence of colors, as in the formation of the color black. When an animal shelter's black dogs are overlooked by prospective adopters, they are rendered invisible. The "excess of black bile" that produces depression is an excess output of the engines of invisibility. The differences between "I" and "we," between the

Asian and the American, between the norm and the model, matter more than ever before even as they cease to matter. Should we be surprised when, among pharmaceutical treatments, one antidepressant is a stimulant that suppresses appetite while another is a calmative that may enhance appetite? Depending on our medications we may lose or gain weight, feel wakeful or drowsy, resigned to celibacy or mad to fornicate. A doctor told me that one of his patients gained one hundred pounds on a prescribed antidepressant but insisted on still taking it because it was easing his depression. Relieved of his melancholy, the patient became newly visible.

We can hardly wonder that depression is called an invisible disability by those who regard it as a disability at all. Racism, as an expression of personal prejudice, is a crime of visibility: a social and political crime. But it is in its institutional form that racism most easily becomes invisible. Any teacher of introductory Ethnic Studies knows the miseries of teaching a definition of institutional racism. Students are familiar with visible signs of prejudice, but glass ceilings are by their very definition invisible. The forces of unequal education, denial of adequate health care, and racial profiling are invisible too. What then must we make of the person of color who is depressed by racism?

Anne Anlin Cheng suggests that racism is not only a source of depression but is also a kind of depression in itself, hence her title: *The Melancholy of Race*. The focus of Cheng's study is the effect of racism on the psyche of the individual sufferer:

> Though a difficult topic and thus rarely discussed, the social and subjective formations of the so-called racialized or minority subject are intimately tied to the psychical experience of grief. This psychical experience is not separate from the realms of society or law but is the very place where the law and society are processed. Even as racism actualizes itself through legal and social sanctions, it is *animated* through imaginative procedures. ... We need to take on the task of acknowledging racial grief in a theoretically and socially responsible way. A sustained focus on the intangible wounds that form the fissures underneath visible phenomena of discrimination should be taking place *in addition to*, not in the place of, the work of advocacy. (original emphasis, Cheng 2001, p. x)

I often explain to students that we have been taught to see episodes of personal prejudice, of a kind that only flagrant bigots enact, *because* they are private and visible, while racist institutional policies are invisible *because* they are public. I discourage students from focusing on the practices of those flagrant bigots as the principal source of racism. What we do not study—what the field of Ethnic Studies generally fails to study—are the effects on mental health of any kind of racism on the individual person of color. This is one of the gaps that Cheng aims to fill.

Most of our narratives of resistance spring from narratives of empowerment. But resistance is made urgent and necessary only because empowerment is elusive. The relationship between the amount of needed resistance and the amount of real empowerment is inverse. If we already had power, we would not be marginalized and would need no resistance. The self-help industry is built on narratives of the personal empowerment of disempowered people, but such narratives of "rags to riches" have no hope of achieving communal justice. Rather than dwell on personal empowerment, scholars of race must build narratives of resistance that examine both communal injustice and the sufferings of individual victims. Cheng argues that personal sufferings are almost impossible to quantify and thus resist the attention of scholars of race, but such neglect is also surely due to the stigma attached to mental illness. If people of color suffer depression, can we hope to mount effective resistance? Cheng suggests that resistance is possible only after we acknowledge and study depression in racialized populations. She even argues that the elements of such study are already available:

> [T]he politics of race has always spoken in the language of psychology. The lesson of psychoanalysis speaks above all to the possibility that *intrasubjectivity exists as a form of intersubjectivity* and that *intersubjectivity often speaks in the voice of intrasubjectivity*: a mutually supportive system. A progressive politics that does not recognize the place of subjective complicity can only be shortsighted. (original emphasis, Cheng 2001, p. 28)

A professor of literature, Cheng might be expected to value the study of subjectivities. Ethnic Studies is usually categorized as a social science, though most work in the field is not quantitative. And yet scholars of race often examine subjectivities only when they examine the cultural productions of racialized peoples. The experience of grief and melancholy may not be a taboo topic, but as with the broader area of physical disabilities, most scholars in the field avoid it.

* * *

I have sought here to ponder the implications of depression in depressed persons of color. A Japanese American diagnosed with severe depression, I have frequently felt isolated in my university—though working in a field whose scholars presume to know how to talk about racism but who seldom consider the sources and effects of depression. I have noticed that people in the field, even when they believe the personal is political, avoid the personal except among close friends. Teaching literature, I notice that students respond intelligently to the ways in which poets such as Adrienne Rich and Audre Lorde and prose writers such as Carlos Bulosan and Toni Morrison read the politics in what Henri Lefebvre calls 'everyday life.' The grief and melancholy of racism are all over books such as *Beloved* (1987) and *America is in the Heart* (1946). Assigning these books, we must continue to teach the social injustices of slavery and dispossession and xenophobia, but we must also ask students to examine the psychical effects of these injustices on individual victims. It is my hope that teaching about depression may encourage depressed students of color to realize that they do not suffer alone, that writers such as Bulosan share the experience and use it as a motivating force toward activism. Communally achieved justice promises an end to privately endured depression.

I have noticed too that, after a semester's instruction in introductory Ethnic Studies, it is usually attentive white students who express hopelessness for the future of race relations. For years I told introductory students that I felt optimistic for the long-term future, that white supremacy would make a last desperate stand before falling. But though Ethnic Studies has existed in the United States for a half-century and more people are more educated about race than ever before, Donald Trump is still elected president, and hate group activity is not only more widespread but also more brashly violent, and so the stand that white supremacy is taking may be desperate but no longer seems like a last one.

My own depression originates mostly from the fallout of my parents' failed relationship, but I will note here two recent sources in my professional life. In 2006, College Republicans staged a hateful anti-immigrant demonstration in the middle of campus, in full view of Ethnic Studies faculty offices. Their president willfully twisted my charges of their xenophobia and racism into an act of profane name-calling, whereupon she demanded my firing. In defense of the College Republicans, the university's "human rights" office ruled that xenophobic hate speech is protected by the administration and that I had violated that protection. In 2015,

Fox News complained that my multicultural literature syllabus, in a line urging all students to defer to the experiences of people of color, threatened coercion to "certain students"—"certain" being code for hostile and white. Because I relate all details of this episode elsewhere, I will offer here those that are pertinent to my argument (Streamas 2019). The dean and provosts ordered me to change the word "deferring," though the dictionary supported my usage, though I had used the word for several years with several classes and no one had complained, and though I was asking all students to "defer" to the "experiences" of people of color rather than to the people themselves, such as those narrated in our literary texts. Shortly after this, I suffered an episode of amnesia and then three months of suicidal thoughts, and afterward I took a Medical Leave of Absence. In both 2006 and 2015 I received racist voicemails and emails, including a few threats: one from a man who claimed to know where I lived and wanted to "see" me. I reported these to the university, even forwarded the most violently racist emails to the dean, but received not even an acknowledgment, much less a message of encouragement, or support, or a promise to defend me.

Depression may involve pain so private that sufferers feel too embarrassed to seek help. But when those sufferers are people of color, and when their reticence owes to a distrust of a system managed by whites, that seems even to be unaware of the most personal effects of racism, then those sufferers are doubly damaged: first by the source of their original pain, and then by the usually indifferent, racist system. Partly because depression remains for all victims insufficiently understood and thus difficult to treat, it is for people of color—for Iris Chang, Kai Cheng Thom, Yiyun Li, and for me—a set of seemingly irreconcilable opposites: real and metaphorical, exceptional and ambient, social and intensely personal.

References

Asianfail. Urban Dictionary. https://www.urbandictionary.com/define.php?term=asian+fail&utm_source=search-action. Accessed 29 December 2017.

Cheng, Anne Anlin. 2001. *The Melancholy of Race: Psychoanalysis, Assimilation, and Hidden Grief*. Oxford: Oxford University Press.

Hopkins, Randy. 2017. Nanjing Echo: Illusion, Subterfuge and Public Relations in the 'Rape of Nanking' Debate, 17 November. www.irischang.net/publications/Nanjing%20Echo%2011-17-2017%20(new%20concl).pdf. Accessed 28 November 2017.

Kamen, Paula. 2007. *Finding Iris Chang: Friendship, Ambition, and the Loss of an Extraordinary Mind*. Philadelphia: Da Capo.

Keevak, Michael. 2011. *Becoming Yellow: A Short History of Racial Thinking*. Princeton, NJ: Princeton University Press.

Lee, S., H.-S. Juon, G. Martinez, C.E. Hsu, E.S. Robinson, J. Bawa, and G.X. Ma. 2009. Model Minority at Risk: Expressed Needs of Mental Health by Asian American Young Adults. *Journal of Community Health* 34 (April): 144–152.

Li, Yiyun. 2017. *Dear Friend, From My Life I Write to You in Your Life*. New York: Random House.

Meyers, Laurie. 2006. Asian-American Mental Health. *Monitor on Psychology* 37 (2) (February): 44. www.apa.org/monitor/feb06/health.aspx.

Preston, Joshua. 2013. The History of the 'Black Dog' as Metaphor. *A Prairie Populist*. https://jppreston.com/2013/09/21/the-history-of-the-black-dog-as-metaphor/.

Price, Margaret, and Stephanie L. Kerschbaum. 2017. *Promoting Supportive Academic Environments for Faculty with Mental Illnesses: Resource Guide and Suggestions for Practice*. Temple University Collaborative (January). www.tuc ollaborative.org. Accessed 28 November 2017.

Schulz, Kirk. 2017a. News and Notes, 29 September. Office of the President. Washington State University. https://president.wsu.edu/2017/09/29/goals-we-will-aspire-to-achieve/. Accessed 28 November 2017.

———. 2017b. News and Notes, 23 October. Office of the President. Washington State University. https://president.wsu.edu/2017/10/23/balancing-the-budget-requires-compromise-sacrifice/. Accessed 28 November 2017.

Solomon, Andrew. 2015. *The Noonday Demon: An Atlas of Depression*, Rev. ed. New York: Scribner.

Streamas, John. 2019. How We Lost Our Academic Freedom: Difference and the Teaching of Ethnic and Gender Studies. In *Teaching with Tension: Race, Resistance, and Reality in the Classroom*, ed. Philathia Bolton, Cassander L. Smith, and Lee Bebout, 143–162. Evanston, IL: Northwestern University Press.

Thom, Kai Cheng. 2016. Belief in Mental Health. *Asian American Literary Review* 7 (2) (Fall/Winter): 4–12.

Ty, Eleanor. 2017. *Asianfail: Narratives of Disenchantment and the Model Minority*. Urbana, IL: University of Illinois Press.

Waldman, Katy. 2014. Black Dog Syndrome. *Slate*, 29 June. www.slate.com/art icles/health_and_science/science/2014/06/black_dog_syndrome_are_peo ple_racist_against_black_pets.html. Accessed 30 November 2017.

Wu, Cynthia. 2016. Diversity Work. *Asian American Literary Review* 7 (2) (Fall/Winter): 40–42.

CHAPTER 5

Blue Histories: Thinking with Sadness in the Middle Ages

Jes Battis

This essay is about feeling sad in the Middle Ages, both as literary convention and readerly response. It is about what Eileen Joy calls a "blue ecological aesthetic" in this literature, a formative sadness (2013, p. 215). In this discussion, I reflect on the relationship between medieval literature and depression, as well as the ways in which reading and teaching this literature has proven therapeutic to me. My literary examples mostly come from the Early Middle Ages, with special attention to the elegy as well as to the wolf in Old English poetry as a companion for difficult times. I approach this topic as a queer, nonbinary and neurodivergent person whose research combines medieval literature and disability studies, as well as someone who has been medicated at various times for anxiety and depression. I'm a wreck in the sense of already having fallen apart, like the ruins in the eponymous Old English poem. Being a wreck led me to medieval literature, while at the same time, it allowed me to see what ruins can offer.

J. Battis (✉)
University of Regina, Regina, SK, Canada

J. Hollenbach and R. A. McDonald (eds.), *Re/Imagining Depression*,
https://doi.org/10.1007/978-3-030-80554-8_5

Old English literature, in particular, has a vein of sadness running through it. Characters wander alone through hostile landscapes. They encounter Roman ruins and cities that have fallen apart, while they are also falling apart, falling out of precarious communities and roaming what was called "Middle-Earth." In the broadest sense, Original Sin was a cause for sadness: life beyond the Garden of Eden was full of harsh knowledge and toil that couldn't replace divine acceptance. Looking back on early medieval literature, Christian writers also felt an ache of sadness for ancient lives that existed outside a framework of grace. The *Beowulf* poet, whoever they were, felt a mixture of curiosity and regret for the Geatish culture that suffuses the poem—the same way most adult writers might discuss their melancholy childhood. When I teach the elegies in particular, students are often surprised by their inherent sadness. But there's also something liberating about feeling blue: the poems offer no "cure" for being incomplete, because the world itself is incomplete. Sadness is a precondition for society.

What is the value in teaching sad, remote literature from a thousand years ago? Part of the goal lies in showing that it isn't so remote. Students are able to recognize the volatile emotional states presented in poems like "The Wife's Lament," or the anxiety of a wizard like Merlin within the Arthurian stories. They sympathize with exiled characters who lack family ties or social supports, because contemporary life can feel that way as well. Self-help culture is obsessed with compulsory happiness, and what Robert McRuer has described as "compulsory able-bodiedness," but this literature refuses any attempts to cure sadness or anxiety (2002, p. 89). In this way, its moodiness can be valuable to an audience dealing with digital cultures and connections that expose their feelings in profound ways. Something very old can be surprisingly useful for negotiating the *now* of our lives.

My first brush with medieval literature was *King Arthur and His Knights*, the nineteenth-century children's version written by James Knowles. I felt—even at nine years old—that I was not the child for whom it had been written. I did not want to be a knight, though I did spend hours pondering Louis Rhead's drawing of Merlin and his crow. The hardcover, with its illustration of an Arthurian twink pulling the sword from the stone, had pride of place next to my *Sword and Sorcery* gaming novels. It was soothing to position their lime green spines in a perfect tower, with the gold dusted special editions at the top. I was just an ordinary kid world-building in their closet while the tabby twined in and out of the map, defining borders with her tail. Years later, a fantasy author would tell me that queer people were all lone wizards. This would have been a useful thing to know as I stared at Merlin through the eyes of that crow, wondering what came next.

A friend and medievalist colleague once described Old English scholars as "crazy." The tone was playful, but the ableist subtext was clear: how could anyone in their so-called "right mind" choose *Beowulf* over *The Canterbury Tales*? Who would eschew the glorious Romance tradition in favor of poems about bloody trees and wolf pups dragged through woods? Later medieval literature has more recognizable structures, like chivalry and aristocracy—anyone who's seen an episode of *Game of Thrones*, or read an Arthurian story, will likely have a sense of how knights and queens may have functioned in the past. But early medieval literature deals with a fragmented "England," divided into at least seven kingdoms and multiple languages. The "English" that we speak today is mostly based on the West Saxon dialect, though we could have easily ended up speaking Kentish or Midlands English, if these dialects had become more far-reaching. The idea of a unified, "Anglo-Saxon" England has been proven to be a racist fiction, designed to buttress the white supremacy that was on the rise in the nineteenth century, and which still seethes today. In reality, early medieval England was a palimpsest of cultures and languages, and Dorothy Kim has argued that medievalists like J. R. R. Tolkien popularized an "an aesthetic, non-politicized, close reading" of early medieval texts like *Beowulf*—a white-centric view that has discriminated against BIPOC medieval scholars in the field (2019, n.p.).

Our stereotype of early medieval literature is men with swords, dying on a battlefield. But much of Old English and Latin writing was deeply concerned with mentality, emotional states, and the effects of loneliness. One of the Old English words for mind is *mod*, and the *mod* trembles across various meanings: in Leslie Lockett's words, it "whistl[es]...like a boiling tea kettle" (2011, p. 70). The *mod* endures lessons and struggles, it plays chess, broods in caves, and rests somewhere between the brain and the heart. In his essay on early medieval psychology, M. R. Godden notes that "*mod* seems to convey to many Anglo-Saxon writers ... something more like an inner passion or willfulness" (1985, p. 287). Lockett also points out that early medieval anatomy located "the mind's activity within the chest cavity," essentially boiling in emotional broth (2011, p. 54). I get it. I was drawn to Old English literature because of what it kept secret; the dark intimacy and drama of being stuck on opposing islands, or forgotten in a cave somewhere, having to build your own world out of fragments.

My mother gave me the Middle Ages. Her childhood was both suffocating and non-traditional, a clash between domestic servitude and hours spent reading and painting. She grew up in a farm town in British Columbia, known for its churches and sweet corn. She came of age in the early fifties: her grandparents still had an outhouse, and her mother was already working in the local cannery as a teenager. At six years old, my mother was the keeper of her younger siblings. My grandmother was full of rage and quick to attack, while my grandfather encouraged reading and serious play. An electrician, he built an electrical panel that controlled every light switch in the house. When my mother had read too long past her bedtime, he'd gently flick her lights off and on. She read Viking sagas about kings named "Bluetooth" and "Gorm the Old." I imagine her beneath the covers—like a manicule in a medieval manuscript, that pointing finger, separating her sisters' beds—while Grendel un-bolted the bone chambers of Hrothgar's men. My father is a polymath, but it was clearly my mother who gave me the medieval gene. She passed it down like the celestial hazelnut given to the medieval mystic Julian of Norwich, which God tells her contains "all that is made" (Norwich 1997, p. 227). An entelechy, or seed, for the whole universe.

I've routinely heard Old English literature described as depressing (the technical adjective is "elegiac," but do these not often amount to the same thing?). An elegy is designed to move its audience from one emotional state to another. Anne Klinck describes the Old English elegy as being preoccupied with "exile, loss of loved ones, scenes of desolation, the transience of worldly joys" (1992, p. 11). Even the accentual metre involves disruption; in *The Ode Less Traveled*, for example, Stephen Fry describes the stresses on either side of the hemistich as "bang and bang … bang and crash," and Ronald Ganze has argued that the speaker in "The Wife's Lament" actually "exhibit[s] the characteristics of Post-Traumatic Stress Disorder" and that this is reflected in her narrative form (Fry 2005, p. 99; Ganze 2015, p. 214). Sadness may not always be the focus of early medieval literature, but it often prevails as a mood, like the subjunctive mood in Old English: a grammatical feeling that drifts away from the concrete, into the dark spaces between islands. Sadness may be a bridge for entering into these works.

When teaching medieval literature, instructors (myself included) often apologize for its difficulty. How many times have I assured students that

Chaucer is "*actually hilarious*," that his bubbling irony is worth the price of learning Middle English? I lure them in with "The Parliament of Fowls", a poem in which flocks of birds debate the nature of love. A duck *quacks* in rhyme royal—what's not to like? But the poem also makes some deeply melancholy observations about human existence: "The lyf so short, the craft so long to lerne ... [The] dredful joy alwey that slit so yerne" (97; L1–2). As they translate together, my students are a bit jolted by the charge of sadness within these lines. Just as the poetic narrator is getting on with his dream vision, he is waylaid by the desire to define dreams—an insomniac outsider looking in. His restless thoughts culminate in a blue stanza:

> The wery hunter slepinge in his bed
> To wode ageyn his minde goth anoon;
> The juge dremeth how his plees been sped;
> The carter dremeth how his cartes goon. (Lynch 2007, p. 99)

> [The weary hunter, sleeping in his bed
> For brighter woods his mind must ever yearn;
> The judge remembers how his pleas were sped
> The carter wonders how his wheels should turn.] (Author's translation)

It's the carter that gets me, like a mechanic dreaming of oil changes. How does the dreamscape frame our lives? Are we ill-equipped to abandon the material of our days, or do we return to it, endlessly, with pleasure? These lines flirt with the idea of escape, while never quite attaining the necessary momentum. Ultimately, they leave me unsatisfied.

I wrote my dissertation on medievalist fiction—that is, fantasy-themed texts that were in conversation with medieval histories and concepts. While exploring queer revisions of the knight in Chaz Brenchley's *Outremer* saga, I fell in love with chivalric manuals: handbooks for transforming a boy into a knight. I was captivated by Geoffroi de Charny's description of the knighting ceremony, which involved far more nudity than I'd anticipated. He cites all the pleasures that a knight's body must avoid, including "the sauce of the court ... [and] choice morsels," suggesting a forbidden chivalric space where knights lounge in feather beds and stall in their transition from soft to hard (1996, p. 111). Giles of Rome was also concerned with the softness of boys, and in his thirteenth century *Regimine principium* (translated by John of Trevisa), he warns that "molles" [soft boys] are "sone ouercome" [soon overcome] (1997,

p. 106). Trevisa uses the Latin word *molles*, from which we derive the term *molly*, an adjective for "softness" that stretches back to the poetry of Martial and Catullus. The task of knighthood is to make the soft hard; to knead dough into steel. In her article on medieval battlefield emotions, Katie Walter identifies this process of making or becoming sad: "The natural heat and softness of a boy's body needs to be tempered by the cold, or be *saddened* … [in] order to become a knight" (2014, p. 26). The Middle English verb *saddened* means to harden, which is precisely what sadness can feel like. Trevisa describes a baking process that ends in cooling: "Colde fastneth the lymes and membres and maken hem sad, so that thei ben the more able to do dedes of armes" [cold fastens the limbs and members of the body, making them hard, so that they are more able to do deeds of arms] (1997, p. 238; author's translation).

School is also a saddening process, by which I mean it is designed to harden us, and that that process of hardening can create despair. As a Master's student, I failed to write a thesis on *Sir Gawain and the Green Knight*. It wasn't a spectacular failure, but rather a daily humiliation that culminated in a desperate message left on my supervisor's answering machine. "I can't do this," I said, while sitting on a couch that was covered in journal articles, some of which had been written in the nineteenth century. At the time, I was living in a bug-infested apartment in Burnaby with three other graduate students who had sensibly decided to study Geography. A colony of spiders had formed in the unsettling gap between the front door and the lintel, and I watched them weaving until I heard the beep of his answering machine. I told him the truth: that the poem was haunting me and yet I had absolutely nothing to say about it. In *The Queer Art of Failure*, J. Halberstam notes that failure can be a sort of style: "Under certain circumstances failing, losing, forgetting, unmaking … [may] in fact offer more creative, more cooperative, more surprising ways of being in the world" (2011, p. 3). I've discussed and criticized this theory of liberatory failure with queer and trans friends, who have experienced the real consequences of failing to conform in a society that would rather we not exist. But Halberstam's "potential" of failure also holds a kind of living space for experimentation and change. In some ways, valuing failure was what propelled me to teach this poem, and eventually—once I'd been hardened—to write about it.

As an undergraduate, I was drawn to Middle English and Icelandic literature, but something about Old English scared me off; the whole corpus seemed to have caution-tape around it. I'd read *Beowulf* in high school, where my English Teacher, Miss Morris, taught us the rudiments of Old and Middle English. She had not appreciated my queer reading of John Knowles's *A Separate Peace* (marking it simply as *too speculative*) and this early reader's report seems to have eclipsed my memories of Old English. In grad school, I encountered the poem "Wulf and Eadwacer" and it felt like swimming in the deep end for the first time. It appears in the Exeter Book, which suggests that it might be a riddle, and was first anthologized by Benjamin Thorpe in 1842 who failed to translate it, saying: "Of this I can make no sense" (as quoted in Malone 1962, p. 107). What medieval scholars know is that "Wulf and Eadwacer" is a poem about three, possibly four, people: Wulf, Eadwacer, an unnamed lord, and a wretched pup. The speaker, distant from Wulf, mourns the loss of days when they were together while fearing what their reunion might precipitate, and the traditional reading suggests a love triangle between an unnamed female speaker and two men. W. J. Sedgefield has also suggested that the speaker might be "a female dog of romantic temperament [who] is dreaming, day-dreaming perhaps, of a wolf with whom she has actually had, or dreams she had, a love affair in the course of her rambles through the forest" (1931, p. 74). No consensus exists on whether the poem's actors are human or canine.

The version of "Wulf and Eadwacer" that I studied was glossed by Harvey De Roo on a neatly typed page with a blue cover. Perhaps because of this, I've always associated the poem with a blue sensibility, what Eileen Joy identifies as a stormy affect concerned with "crumbling persons, crumbling worlds" (2013, p. 215). So many Old English poems are about worlds that seem to have already fallen apart: ruins, empty hoards, broken families. The people in elegies are "crumbling," to quote Joy, as they struggle to deal with the blue strains of sadness, dislocation, and regret. In an early medieval world that was only loosely connected by communities and hearths, like small points of life, the scariest thing was to be alone, unrooted, in that map-less blue space. When I was a grad student, I rented a seventies apartment with shag carpeting and a very blue room: it featured a blue velvet *fleur-de-lis* decoration that my ex-boyfriend called "the mural." After we broke up, I remember staring at the mural as if it were somehow responsible. The truth was that we'd both failed quite exceptionally at being good for one another, which made the end feel as natural as a line break. The apartment had seen an endless series of roommates that included an exotic dancer, a man who didn't sleep, and a student whose cat routinely shit on my pillow. My failure to translate a twelve-hundred year old poem with no clear pronouns seemed fairly benign when considered in this context.

"Wulf and Eadwacer" ends with a moment of dazzling opacity, a failure to convey clear meaning, when the speaker calls out to Eadwacer:

> Gehyrest þu, Eadwacer? Uncerne earne hwelp
> bireð Wulf to wuda.
> þæt mon eaþe tosliteð þætte næfre gesomnad wæs,
> uncer giedd geador. (Muir 1994, p. 286)

> [Eadwacer, do you hear? Wulf
> drags our whelp to the woods.
> Men simply shred what was never sound,
> our [ ] together.] (Author's translation)

The noun "giedd" means song, lay, riddle, poem, and speech—nothing that can physically be split apart. Does the speaker refer to a sack that Wulf drags behind him, enclosing the body of a poor pup? How could this "Eadwacer" [Dawn-Watcher] hear what Wulf is doing? David Clark links the word "earmne" [wretched] to a state of sexual exile and reads the whelp as queer: "A young man … [imprisoned] on an island and socially ostracized for engaging in a sexual relationship with another man, Wulf" (2009, p. 30). In this reading, the whelp becomes a queer cub dragged into exile, with "giedd" signifying a forbidden relationship. Victoria Blud takes this sly reading to task for stressing "[the] precariousness of the female character—by writing her out of the poem altogether" (2014, p. 342). As a (hopefully) productive middle ground, I'd like to suggest that both Clark and Blud are right. Erasing women from the poem is certainly not the answer, but neither is assuming that the speaker is female-bodied, or even cisgender. Instead, the speaker's voice can play with grammatical gender, becoming trans or nonbinary, while offering a refrain that is queer in its citation of radical difference: "ungelic is us" [we are different]. In his contemporary poem about "Wulf and Eadwacer" (using the same title), Miller Oberman describes the indeterminacy of the work as being open in the most inclusive sense:

> And when it ["giedd"] disappears
> who is to say then what it meant,
> what form it had, whose mouth
> released it thoughtlessly. (2017, p. 8)

These productive uncertainties within "Wulf and Eadwacer" keep me tethered to it; I can't seem to break up with this poem. I teach it whenever I can, letting students fill in the blanks however they choose. Like so many experiences that are ultimately untranslatable, it invites what José Esteban Muñoz calls "practiced failure," which contains "a certain mode of virtuosity" (2009, pp. 183, 173). When you can't succeed, you can always fail in a fabulous register.

I had wolves on the mind when I fell apart—not for the first time, but perhaps more publicly than ever before. I had just completed my comprehensive exams, which involved reading for hours every day, until migraines dug a garden in my skull. I often went to a Starbucks located in the Pacific Centre Mall, because they allowed me to stay and work uninterruptedly for long periods of time. My reading companion most days was a monk with whom I never exchanged a single word. He wore dark Fluevogs, and we were able to be "alone with each other" (Byatt 2011, p. 471). After passing the exams and defending my wobbly thesis prospectus, something in me splintered. I refused to do anything that I was asked. I ate nothing but Glico curry while watching *Six Feet Under*, convinced that I'd entered a dream-vision. A friend told me that I was acting "like a robot." I didn't mention that I'd also stopped using the couch, and was treating the floor as a surface appropriate to all occasions. I napped with the cat, dreaming of the giant wolf from *The Neverending Story*. Though he had failed to kill the boy-warrior Atreyu, he succeeded in scaring the shit out of me when I first saw him on a 25-foot movie screen. I told my mother that I was dreaming of wolves, and she tactfully suggested that I might want to come home for a bit. This trip resulted in my introduction to Prozac, a drug that I took for eight years. There was something inescapably medieval about it.

A drug like Prozac tells the brain to release all of its serotonin, like Beowulf liberating the dragon's hoard. This does not result in a tingling sensation of wellbeing; for the first month that I took it, I existed in a drowned state from which I could barely form sentences. I remember sitting in a Tim Horton's with my parents, unable to follow a thought to completion. I stared at my coffee like it was a *giedd*, a riddle-object, whose purpose eluded me so completely that it must have been some unearthed fragment. My mother handed me my cup, as if she were handing me the medieval world. I thought of Queen Wealtheow in *Beowulf*, who controls the cup, and therefore the feast in miniature. She decides who drinks first, who will be honored. That's her role as a "fríþwebba", or "peace-weaver." My mother was trying to weave peace in my mind.

The early medieval poetic record is full of self-help literature, by which I mean guides to life written in the absence of a unified method. The eighth-century monk and scholar, Alcuin, was forever asking for books in his correspondence, guarding them jealously, searching for theories. He describes the act of writing sorrow as "[d]ipping my loving pen in a sea of tears" (Allott 1974, p. 146). Since his beloved Arno (Bishop of Salzburg) wouldn't see his face, he might instead read the textual affect in its place. He worried about his young charges moving alone through the world, calling them dear animals. What would they get up to in the taverns of Italy? Some of the instructional Old English poems, like "Maxims" [1-C], read as apocalyptic road literature. You get the sense of exiles tracking you throughout the poem, keeping pace with you in the shadows just beyond the path. This path is both literal, in the sense of a navigable road, and symbolic, a common knowledge-bond shared by those following in each other's footsteps across Middle Earth. Reconciliation of exile is the preoccupation of "Maxims" and, queerly, the exile's companion in this poem is also a wolf. In "Maxims", the wolves often slink out of formulaic verses meant to describe battlefield carnage. Sometimes they wait greedily for human failure. In *Maxims*, I argue, they take on the role of anti-companion to the exile, the opposite of friendly road-mate:

> Wineleas, wonsælig mon genimeð him wulfas to geferan,
> felafæcne deor. Ful oft hine se gefera sliteð;
> gryre sceal for greggum, græf deadum men;
> hungre heofeð, nales þæt heafe bewindeð,
> ne huru wæl wepeð wulf se græga,
> morþorcwealm mæcga, ac hit a mare wille. (Muir 1994, p. 257)

> [The friendless, ill-fated man / wanders, wolf-companion,
> with sly wildfellows. Too often they bite the fellowship;
> He should fear the graylings, / dig ditches for the dead;
> Wulf sings for hunger, / but that high, binding cry
> is no threnody for slaughter / that grey one,
> mourns not the quelled dead / but howls for more.] (Author's translation)

Here the wolf sings the end of humanity. Wolves den in the ruins of the Anthropocene, yet while civilization persists, they keep their human companions' company. As mourners, they seduce us towards blue places, inspiring what Eileen Joy describes as "a willingness to draw close to the sadness of others" (2013, p. 226). The unexpected presence of the wolf in this poem can also be a comfort. The exile is never alone: the wolf fares with them along this alien path. There is a witness to all this grave digging. I was once at a conference on medieval ecologies and a participant asked what we might do to help reverse the human-driven extinction event known as the Anthropocene. A presenter responded: "We can die." Nervous laughter rippled through the audience, but this is the wolf's maxim as well. Death remains the exile's choice, fraught as it may be with the sin of despair. Judas and Cain, the original exiles, form a geneaology of *desperatio* [despair] in Old English literature. In his work on medieval suicide, Alexander Murray defines *desperatio* as "a failure to hope for God's mercy" (2000, p. 377). In Old English vernacular literature, this becomes the failure to admit a sense of worldedness; a turning away from kith and kin. The exile is both "acolmod" [cold-minded] and, conversely, full of burning anxiety. In her work on early medieval psychologies, Leslie Lockett describes the "hydraulic" model of emotions, where feelings begin in the pressure cooker of the chest. They eventually burst out like "a tea kettle full of boiling water, whistling" (2011, p. 70). The exile whistles and the wolf answers.

I use Old English poetry in the classroom as a means of talking about anxiety and depression. We discuss the seafarer, alone on the water, perhaps locked in his own mind and inseparable from the "isigfeþera" [frost-locked] feathers of the seabirds (Muir 1994, p. 233). Students are particularly curious about "The Wife's Lament", a poem that Ronald Ganze identifies with trauma, explaining that the speaker's "traumatic experiences have … [so] affected her ability to encode and retrieve memories that what remains of her experience are a few, scattered details" (2015, p. 224). We discuss the common anxieties felt by wanderers—uncertainty, loss of friends and family support—as well as the highly specific anxieties that only the wanderer can understand. This intimate knowledge is crucial to the poem's presentation of sadness, as well as the agency of the sad person for whom something always remains untranslatable, and wherein individual sadness resists general diagnosis. We compare "The Wife's Lament" to Virginia Woolf's suicide note, in which she expresses painful agency: "I am doing what seems the best thing to do … I don't think two people could have been happier than we have been." The speaker in "The Wife's Lament" asserts a similar agency:

> Ic þis giedd wrece / bi me ful geomorre,
> minre sylfre sið. (Muir 1994, p. 331)

> [I will weave this self-song / my own mourning,
> in my own words.] (Author's translation)

We discuss the self that emerges from sadness, how it resists interpretation as an indeclinable noun. This is a literature that attends to depression, that lingers over instability and a feeling of restlessness. In the *Medieval Disability Studies Sourcebook*, Cameron Hunt McNabb links "medieval" with "disability" as similarly contested terms: "The term 'disability' presents complexities similar to 'the Middle Ages,' including under its umbrella disabilities marked as physical, emotional, and mental; chronic and acute; visible and invisible" (2020, p. 13). By discussing medieval writing in and through a disability studies framework, students are able to think through the history of emotions, to think with sadness, as these poets may have done.

As Jay Dolmage notes in *Academic Ableism*, the structure of academia—with its relentless focus on production and professional comportment—"powerfully mandates able-bodiedness and able-mindedness, as well as other forms of social and communicative hyperability, and this demand can best be defined as ableism" (2017, p. 7). His description of "communicative hyperability" is particularly resonant with me, since, in spite of my vocabulary and training as an educator, I often struggle to communicate verbally—especially under pressure. But medieval studies can actually help with this, since dealing with issues of translation and historical analysis can open up space for discussing how we read and process difficult texts. Coming out as disabled in the classroom is no single, uniform act. There is no simple disclosure, and Alison Kafer notes that the act of coming out can even be triggering to others: "My talk *itself* might change the space, making it no longer habitable—or habitable only under certain conditions—to some audience members" (2016, p. 3).

When I was in college, a psychology professor informed the class that they were taking anti-depressants. When they did, they did so with a decided change in tone, suggesting that this was not a casual admission, but rather a measured and difficult confession. I remember how surprised I was (and later, how grateful), as if they had pointed out an invisible door. I realize now that they were an adjunct instructor at the time, so their admission was even more dangerous due to lack of job security. In my classes on queer literature and history, I come out right away as both queer and gender-queer: it may seem effortless in the moment, but it was once a Herculean effort, and still bears the marks of past struggle. But when discussing literatures of disability, I'm far more conflicted about performing this "confession." I ask myself: What communities am I invoking? What diagnoses and potentially traumatic histories am I bringing into the room? Peta Cox describes the act of "passing as sane," which "occurs when a person who is experiencing psychological distress or non-normative emotional states or cognition manages to avoid displaying these states in the presence of others" (2013, p. 100). I would say that this roughly describes my daily experience, both in a classroom and within the more broadly ableist structures of academia. I may look comfortable at the front of the classroom, but a part of me—my wanderer—is silently freaking out. Not because of imposter syndrome or the anxiety of public speaking, but because I am *always freaking out*. This is my style.

None of the poems I have discussed so far seek a cure for sadness. They are content to remain within what "Maxims" describes as "deop deada wæg" [the deep dales/deadways] (Bjork 2014, p. 70). There is no cure because sadness is part of the world rather than a temporary state. This allows for a consideration of ideologies of cure often mobilized against disabled and neurodivergent people, and how one response might be to carve out living space within one's particular failure to be "normal." Like Old English emotional states, our contemporary emotional worlds are resistant to translation. In *Brilliant Imperfection*, Eli Clare notes that "at the center of cure lies eradication and the many kinds of violence that accompany it ... [cure] arrives in many different guises, connected to elimination and erasure in a variety of configurations" (2017, p. 26). An organization like Autism Speaks, for example, wherein no member of the board of directors is autistic, still frames its mandate in terms of "curing" a natural form of neurodiversity. In her 2020 memoir, autistic writer Sarah Kurchak notes that Autism Speaks, "our most prominent charity…assumes that we can't do so for ourselves and therefore appoints itself the savior who can and should assume the responsibility" (2020, n.p.). In order to approach literature within a disability studies framework, we need to privilege the voices of disabled scholars, to explore states of unrest and difference that remain richly uncategorized. Disability in the Middle Ages was not an easily quantifiable experience, and Joshua Eyler notes that while some conflated impairment with sin, "this way of understanding medieval disability has only limited viability. In truth, there were many lenses through which medieval societies viewed disability" (2010, p. 3).

While teaching a class on Medieval women's literature, I began to discuss "The Wife's Lament", a poem about intensities described by an overwhelmed narrator, in relationship to anxiety and environmental sensitivity. The speaker describes a feeling of "uhtceare" [dawn-care], a specific sort of anxiety born in the liminal moment between night and day. At the same time, this is also a particular experience: my own trajectory of depression has always included a troubling relationship with sleep. We know little about this person—even her gender is somewhat fluid, given that we're basing her cis-womanhood on a few feminized Old English adjectives. She's been left somewhere in a sort of cave, where she remembers someone who may have been an old lover. The class was particularly drawn to the speaker's description of stoicism in the face of turmoil—a convention in Old English poetry that seems quite impossible in this situation:

> A scyle geong mon wesan geomormod,
> heard heortan geþoht, swylce habban sceal
> bliþe gebæro, eac þon breostceare,
> sinsorgna gedreag .... (Muir 1994, p. 332)

> [A young person, sorrow-minded,
> must be hard-hearted in thought,
> always seem happy, while mazed by
> a storm of troubles.] (Author's translation)

The Old English *mon* is gender-neutral, so the "geong" [young] "mon" can be anyone. The poem offers ironic advice for suppressing emotions, while still knowing that this performance is doomed to fail. In class, this leads to a discussion of strategies for dealing with anxiety, the pressures of appearing within a classroom, and the shocks of young adulthood that may be compounded by neurodiversity.

It can be liberating to recite, teach, and puzzle over sad literature—to acknowledge that many different minds often have sadness in common. Medieval literature often leads me to Sara Ahmed's question: "Do we consent to happiness?" (2010, p. 1). In *The Promise of Happiness*, Ahmed seeks to challenge what she calls "the idea that we have a responsibility to be happy for others" (2010, p. 9). It has taken me a long time to realize that I cannot shoulder this responsibility, nor should I. Enforced happiness is simply another form of McRuer's "compulsory able-bodiedness ... [the] experience of the able-bodied need for an agreed-on common ground" (2002, pp. 89, 92). Often, happiness is expected within definitions of "collegiality" and can even become part of an academic's performance criteria. It is expected of students in the form of "engagement," while ignoring the fact that students, like faculty, enter classrooms in various states of mental distress. There is also the preposterous notion that instructors will know engagement when we see it, and that criteria designed by neurotypical researchers should apply to neuroatypical students and teachers. In *Mad At School*, Margaret Price argues that "some of the most important common topoi of academe intersect problematically with mental disability," including concepts such as "rationality … participation … [and] collegiality" (2011, p. 5). Price goes on to uncover her own relationship with disability, in an effort of reclamation:

> In naming myself a crazy girl, neuroatypical, mentally disabled, psychosocially disabled—in acknowledging that I appear (as a colleague once told me) 'healthy as a horse' yet walk with a mind that whispers in many voices—I am trying to reassign meaning … [naming] myself pragmatically according to what context requires. (p. 20)

As a writer and scholar, I have found teaching medieval literature to be therapeutic and ultimately helpful in this effort to "reassign meaning." Old English poems, including "Wulf and Eadwacer", "Maxims", and "The Wife's Lament", have allowed me to present a medieval framework for discussing anxiety and depression. My students have also found these distant perspectives to be surprisingly familiar, and wanderers and wolves have offered them an unexpected language for discussing affect and worldly intensity. Leslie Lockett reminds me that "overwhelm," a common word associated with stress and grief, comes from the Old English verb "weallan" [to boil] (2011, p. 59). To be overwhelmed is to boil over, to seethe within the gap between despair and hard-heartedness. Sadness can be an argument that challenges conventional academic rhetoric, whistling in the margins. There are particularly medieval ways for thinking about and through sadness which take us to a critical blue space. For me, this space has been transformative, and has allowed for new thinking within medieval disability studies. Poetry that attends to unstable emotional states and inchoate experiences can reclaim creative strategies for living on a spectrum of disability: wandering, wolfing, lamenting our way into new solidarities and queer definitions. Medieval literature often presents a world in which joy is elusive and sadness is the norm, freeing us from compulsory modes of happiness and giving us permission to feel medieval.

References

Ahmed, Sara. 2010. *The Promise of Happiness*. Durham: Duke University Press.

Allott, Stephen (ed.). 1974. *Alcuin of York: His Life and Letters*. York: William Sessions.

Bjork, Robert E. 2014. *Old English Shorter Poems, Volume One: Wisdom and Lyric*. Cambridge, MA: Harvard University Press.

Blud, Victoria. 2014. Wolves' Heads and Wolves' Tales: Women and Exile in *Bisclavret* and *Wulf and Eadwacer*. *Exemplaria* 26 (4): 328–346.

Byatt, A.S. 2011. *Possession*. New York: Vintage.

Charney, Geffroi. 1996. *The Book of Chivalry*, ed. Richard Kaeuper. Philadelphia: University of Pennsylvania Press.

Clare, Eli. 2017. *Brilliant Imperfection: Grappling with Cure*. Durham: Duke University Press.

Clark, David. 2009. *Between Medieval Men*. Oxford: Oxford University Press.

Cox, Peta. 2013. Passing as Sane, or How to Get People to Sit Next to You on the Bus. In *Disability and Passing: Blurring the Lines of Identity*, ed. Jeffrey Brune, 99–110. Philadelphia: Temple University Press.

Dolmage, Jay. 2017. *Academic Ableism: Disability and Higher Education*. Ann Arbor: University of Michigan Press.

Eyler, Joshua, ed. 2010. *Disability in the Middle Ages: Reconsiderations and Reverberations*. Surrey: Ashgate.

Fry, Stephen. 2005. *The Ode Less Traveled*. London: Hutchinson.

Ganze, Ronald. 2015. The Neurological and Physiological Effects of Emotional Duress on Memory in Two Old English Elegies. In *Anglo-Saxon Emotions*, ed. Alice Jorgensen, 211–226. Surrey: Ashgate.

Godden, M.R. 1985. Anglo-Saxons On the Mind. In *Learning and Literature in Anglo-Saxon England*, ed. Michael Lapidge, 271–298. Cambridge: Cambridge University Press.

Halberstam, J. 2011. *The Queer Art of Failure*. Durham: Duke University Press.

Joy, Eileen. 2013. Blue. In *Prismatic Ecology: Ecotheory Beyond Green*, ed. Jeffrey Jerome Cohen, 213–232. Minneapolis: University of Minnesota Press.

Kafer, Alison. 2016. Un/Safe Disclosures: Scenes of Disability and Trauma. *Journal of Literary and Cultural Disability Studies* 10 (6): 1–20.

Kim, Dorothy. 2019. The Question of Race in *Beowulf*. *JSTOR Daily*. https://daily.jstor.org/the-question-of-race-in-beowulf/.

Klinck, Anne. 1992. *The Old English Elegies: A Critical Edition*. Ottawa: Carleton University Press.

Kurchak, Sarah. 2020. *I Overcame My Autism and All I Got Was This Lousy Anxiety Disorder*. Douglas & McIntyre [Kindle Edition].

Lockett, Leslie. 2011. *Anglo-Saxon Psychologies in the Vernacular and Latin Traditions*. Toronto: University of Toronto Press.

Lynch, Kathryn, ed. 2007. *Dream Visions and Other Poems: Geoffrey Chaucer*. London: W. W. Norton.

Malone, Kemp. 1962. Two English Frauenlieder. *Comparative Literature* 14 (1): 106–117.

McNabb, Cameron Hunt, ed. 2020. *Medieval Disability Sourcebook*. Santa Barbara, CA: Punctum Books.

McRuer, Robert. 2002. Compulsory Able-Bodiedness and Queer/Disabled Existence. In *Disability Studies: Enabling the Humanities*, ed. Sharon Snyder, et al., 88–99. New York: MLA.

Muir, Bernard, ed. 1994. *The Exeter Anthology of Old English Poetry*, vol. 1. Exeter: University of Exeter Press.

Muñoz, José Esteban. 2009. *Cruising Utopia: The Then and There of Queer Futurity*. New York: NYU Press.

Murray, Alexander. 2000. *Suicide in the Middle Ages II: The Curse on Self-Murder*. Oxford: Oxford University Press.

Norwich, Julian. 1997. Shewings. In *The Writings of Medieval Women*, ed. Marcelle Thiébaux, 221–234. Oxford: Garland.

Oberman, Miller. 2017. *The Unstill Ones*. Princeton University Press.

Price, Margaret. 2011. *Mad At School: Rhetorics of Mental Disability and Academic Life*. Ann Arbor: University of Michigan Press.

Sedgefield, W.J. 1931. Old English Notes: *Wulf and Eadwacer*. *Modern Language Review* 26 (1): 74–75.

Trevisa, John (translator). 1997. *The Governance of Kings and Princes*, ed. David Fowler et al. Oxford: Garland.

Walter, Katie. 2014. Peril, Flight and the Sad Man: Medieval Theories of the Body in Battle. *Essays and Studies* 67: 21–40.

CHAPTER 6

Teaching/Depression as a Queer Theory for Living

Alyson Hoy

I completed my PhD eight years ago, not at Duke, but at the University of British Columbia, and yet, I am still, after all this time, Eve Sedgwick's student. Eve Sedgwick was a major figure in queer theory and, indeed, one of the discipline's founding scholars, but she left her imprint on numerous other fields as well, including literary studies, gender studies, affect studies, performance studies, and human geography. She died on April 12, 2009 after living eighteen years with breast cancer. Even today, her work feels like theory for living, beaming a light on the multiple queer pathways and possibilities that exist for thinking, making, being, and living. Throughout my doctoral studies when I was struggling not only with questions about my queerness and what seemed the shifting nature of my sexuality, but also with anorexia, self-harm, and depression, Sedgwick's writing functioned in no small way as sustenance. I do not want to say, absolutely, that I had given up on life at the exact moment in which I should have been anticipating a future, yet, increasingly and with urgency I was looking for the exit sign.

A. Hoy (✉)
University of British Columbia, Vancouver, Canada

J. Hollenbach and R. A. McDonald (eds.), *Re/Imagining Depression*,
https://doi.org/10.1007/978-3-030-80554-8_6

In "Teaching/Depression," an essay that serves in important ways as a departure point for my thinking about the spiralling bout of depression that gripped me during the two years I spent writing my doctoral dissertation, Sedgwick states "there is a lot to say and wonder about the relation between depression, under its many definitions, and the kinds of work we do over the decades as feminists, as intellectuals and activists, as autobiographers, and as teachers" (2006, p. 1). Curious about the potential connections between teaching and depression, Sedgwick links the two implicitly in the essay and, indeed, suggests that they are opposite sides of the same coin with the use of a forward slash in the title. She reminds readers that Silvan Tomkins, when writing about shame, labelled the educator as a "depressive personality" (2006, p. 1) and she proceeds from there to challenge the limitations and contradictions inherent in popular understandings of depression by juxtaposing Tomkins' understanding of "depressiveness" with Melanie Klein's description of a "depressive position." For Sedgwick, the uniqueness and generosity of Klein's account inheres in its understanding of the productive possibilities of the depressive position or the ways that, as a "uniquely spacious rubric," it is "potentially available to everyone" (p. 3), and that it may even be sought out as a resource for surviving, repairing, and moving beyond depression.

Interested less in arriving at a particular understanding of depression or, even, in exploring the intricate and multiple meanings and experiences of depression in different contexts and across life stages, Sedgwick instead attends closely to the idea of relationality. In the essay, she teases out the question: what are the relations between depression, pedagogy, and autobiography? What does it mean to view depression as a "pre-requisite" for a pedagogic/critical practice? (p. 1). For Sedgwick, pedagogy refers to something bigger and more expansive than the academic institution itself. As a mode of relationality, it opens up spaces of possibility where certain types of emotional thinking or work can become available, and where difficult emotions can subsequently be harnessed and made use of in the classroom, in writing, and in life.

To experience grief, despair, and depression is, as Julia Cooper writes in her recent, eloquent study of dying and the art of eulogy, to dwell in the presence of "ugly or artless feelings" (2017, p. 102). Seeking a means by which to explore and engage with grief as opposed to hurrying through it or turning away from it altogether, Cooper locates her project explicitly "in the tradition of Eve Sedgwick" and the "emotional and hopefully healing approach to knowledge ... she championed" (p. 100).

There is a usefulness, a language, and, indeed, a knowledge of suffering that are virtually lost to us, Cooper suggests, in so far as rituals of modern mourning centre on performing but not feeling grief, “a compulsion to rapidly [and publicly] articulate that which is so hard to put into words” (p. 40). At one point she writes, “I wonder if there is a way we might pay homage to the disorientation that loss brings and leave some room to not know what to do in the face of it” (p. 35).

By turns beautifully Sedgwickian, Cooper does just that, making “palpable—and available”—a space within her own process of creating and of writing, allowing readers to wander in and rest for a bit, and then, if we choose, to explore and connect with lingering feelings of sadness (2017, p. 101). Writing is, for Cooper, as it was for Sedgwick, a way of holding our dead and continuing our talks with them. By the same turn, it also serves as a means for reparation and of being held. In what follows, I recount my experiences of depression and anorexia, weaving the critical threads of my PhD dissertation on Sedgwick’s queer reparative theory with vignettes from my memoir writings on sexuality, desire, embodiment, trauma, and emergent queer identities. Bringing into public view and attempting to connect to other histories and accounts of my personal experience of depression, I take up and perform Sedgwick’s method of reparative reading not strictly as an academic inquiry on depression but as she more broadly conceived of and intended it: as a vital resource beyond the classroom and as a queer theory for living.

In my dissertation Sedgwick’s writing and criticism take centre stage, but her work comprises less an object of study requiring a method of reading that is distant, detached, and calculating than it does an apparatus for thinking as playful and pleasurable experimentation. Her work presents a mode of inquiry unable to determine in advance its course, and unafraid, finally, not to know. In a hostile and typically shame-prone environment such as the academy, Sedgwick’s legacy is a model of intellectual exploration that is relentless in its precision and attention. As a queer critical practice her writing enacts an exquisite embodied intimacy, inviting readers to enter into the processes of contingent thought and analysis in a temporality of the present, and confounding and remapping accepted decorum regarding “appropriate” associations between subjects and objects, including the relationship between herself as author, the subject matter of her inquiry, and the reader.

Amongst the considerable and still growing body of critical work dedicated to a careful examination of Sedgwick’s oeuvre, generous is one of the most frequent and enduring descriptions, employed by scholars most commonly to denote the remarkable ways in which her writing explicitly sought to clear intellectual and affective space for others—to grant permission. As Heather Love explains, "reading her work tends to open unexpected conceptual possibilities, ways of thinking, gestures, and tones" (2010, p. 235). Enabling is the word that Love uses to describe Sedgwick's "effect," acknowledging that while "there are so many things [it] could mean," it actually rather fittingly suggests a sense of "opening or enlargement" where readers encounter forms of knowledge and are "pushed—pleasurably—to the limits of what is knowable for them and then over the edge" (p. 235).

For me, this sense of being enabled has been and continues to be an effect of reading and studying Sedgwick, of coming to feel cared for as her student. Sedgwick enabled me—for the first time, really—to see the queer world-making potentialities of my own life. In Sedgwick's prose I found permission to feel confused and to be incoherent in relation to desire. Inspired by the generosity of her writing and how it embraced, as Annamarie Jagose suggests, "things more usually presumed to have nothing to say to each other," I could ask from the depth of my shame whether writing feels like self-harming or like fucking (Jagose 2010, p. 13). I could argue, with respect to anorexia, that what appears on the surface of things as the cruellest, most annihilating impulse to starve and deny and waste the self through racking and incessant hunger and to refuse intimate and interpersonal connection is queerly oriented to life and not only death. I do not mean to suggest that Sedgwick in any way personally or heroically saved me from the brink and reaffirmed my attachment to life, but her theoretical work, more than a mere conduit for thinking, opened up a space for sex and desire that, in countless surprising ways, made me want to want.

Starting from one dictionary definition of resilience as "the ability of an object to return to its usual shape after being bent, stretched, or pressed," I want to attempt to think through the idea of queer resilience by placing it in the context of Sedgwick's theorizing of reparation and the distinctly queer and hopeful method she called reparative reading. Reparative reading is a critical practice that begins from a position of psychic damage—what Sedgwick calls the depressive position—and that bears within it the possibility of a reparative position that picks up the fragments of a sustainable life. Grounded in disillusion rather than infatuation, it arises, as one critic describes, "from the obvious fact that our world is damaged and dangerous" but instead of "repeat[ing] the bad news" it seeks to "build or rebuild some more sustaining [and loving] relation to the objects in our world" (Hanson 2011, p. 103). Reparation is, for Sedgwick, about learning how to create small worlds of sustenance that cultivate a different present and future for the losses that one has suffered. She calls on hope as a critical reparative energy, one that gives the reader "room to realize that [because] the future may be different from the present, it is also possible…to entertain such profoundly painful, profoundly relieving, ethically crucial possibilities as that the past, in turn, could have happened differently too" (2003, p. 143).

I can be brave and say, at the risk of sounding unknowing, that there is something that remains enigmatic about Sedgwick's theorizing of the reparative and depressive position as "[the] position from which it is possible in turn to use one's own resources to assemble or 'repair' the murderous part-objects into something like a whole—though … not necessarily like any pre-existing whole" (2003, p. 128). The difficulty I think stems not just from the density of the language—and, indeed, she does frame it psychoanalytically, which, as a rule, requires its own special kind of decoding—but rather from my own (do I dare say, cynicism?) that any one of us might actually return to the past and from the ruins of personal and historical damage successfully piece together a recognizable self and see a world transformed. The place in her writing where the idea seems the most legible or at least *feels* the most pressing is her theorizing of shame which, via loving excavation and exploration of painful and isolating events from the past, she reactivates and creates anew as a useful, pleasurable, and even joyous affect in the present.

Crucial to queer theorists who over the years have attempted to rethink 'gay pride' and the emotions that surround it, shame in Sedgwick's analysis stunningly escapes tautology such that it yields knowledges not at all equivalent to the sense of shame with which one starts out. Shame and excitement may at first seem incompatible to readers yet viewed through the lens of Sedgwick's discussion of her own queerness or what she describes as the "non-unified multiplicity" of her sexualities, shame breaks almost completely with its conventional associations of negativity and pathology and instead emerges in her text as the very condition of pleasurable possibility (1999, p. 158). Speaking to Shannon, the psychotherapist whose services she seeks and with whom she ultimately though not easily enters into an intimate, loving dialogue across difference as she works to recover from chemotherapy, a mastectomy, and a subsequent spiralling depression, Sedgwick notes that "sexiness and embarrassment are two things that won't ever stay separate for me. It's *exciting* for me to talk about this with him" (1999, p. 171).

In interweaving fantasy and reality—"two, utterly separate worlds"—shame does a lot of work in *A Dialogue on Love*, propelling the narrative forward through the author's own, often perverse, sexualized investment (1999, p. 48). From her near obsessive recollecting of her sexual childhood self, which she narrates to Shannon as the compulsively "masturbating girl," to an account of the S/M fantasies that play out as she gives blood in an examination room during her cancer treatment, to an inquiry into the relationship between art and sex where experimentation with poetic form and the hammering iteration of rhythm recall the erotic charge and trauma of the scene of childhood spanking from her past, Sedgwick interrupts sexuality and, specifically, queer and non-normative sexualities as a primary site for the reproduction of bad feeling. Yet, even beyond her stunning proclivity and talent to do strange things with words, to free shame from pathologizing narratives and queerly transform its contents into raw, unabashed ecstasy, she offers as well, in the very act of speaking about it, an invitation and an incitement to pleasure. In dialogue with her therapist, and addressing the public readers of her private record, Sedgwick writes:

> There's something about pleasure that might be important. I don't know how to say it properly; I've gotten hold of an intuition that if things can change for me, it won't be through a very grim process...I used to take one deep masochistic breath, and determine I was ready to surrender to the disciplinary machine –in enough pain to have to do it –but then of course I didn't know how to, and couldn't sustain my resolve anyway; and nothing about the therapy would work. Now it seems that if anything can bring me through to real change, it may only be some kind of pleasure. (p. 45)

The notion of pleasure, and what needs to be, as Sedgwick's work articulates, the persistent and unapologetically public attempt to prioritize and record and circulate the surprising, multiple queer ways it gets experienced (i.e.., not just as warm, spreading sensation or lust and ecstatic feeling, but as intrinsic to and carefully intertwined with pain and suffering and damage), is the heartbeat of both the reparative mode and a queer ethics and politics. As I have already suggested, it is significant that my capacity to read and think and write, seemingly against all odds, in the midst of illness and trauma and while being inscribed by the debilitating codes of negativity—self-destruction, passivity, masochism—was enabled by Sedgwick's reparative mode. As criticism and a way of knowing that seeks pleasure and enacts care for the self, it mercifully approximates "the work of love" (Britzman 2003, p. 137).

Before Sedgwick, I had been thinking a lot about how lonely and at times dissociating it felt to be engaged in intellectual inquiry and whether the process of coming to know something ought always to involve some kind of pain and destruction –coming undone in proximity to one's object, for example, or cutting a hole in the self so that the thing endured can put down roots. To the extent that her writing held open the possibility of being in some "other" relation to myself, to others, to the academy, and in the meaningful and unparalleled role it played in forming a queer public, it helped to expand my thinking to consider the ways in which so-called 'individual', 'personal', and 'private' experiences of shame and suffering also connect to broader public cultures and collective histories. True to Sedgwick, I did not anticipate how stunning the realization would be, that finally, upon completing my dissertation, the burden was no longer mine alone to carry. I did not know how emptying it would feel to publicly articulate all that was damaged and despairing and ugly in my own life and discover from that, like pebbles rippling in a pond, the quiet, collective reverberations of hope emerged.

The Queer Crush of Intellect

Eve Sedgwick states in "A Poem Is Being Written" that "this essay was written late: twenty-seven years late, to the extent that it represents a claim for respectful attention to the intellectual and artistic life of a nine-year-old child Eve Kosofsky" (1993, p. 177). I did not know that child and yet I feel a certain fierce and indestructible faithfulness to her. Like the gasp that escapes my lungs when the first brightly coloured drops of blood appear, or the awareness, the pulsing, fermenting sensation that feelings of admiration and curiosity about somebody have suddenly become a crush, I want this writing to claim a shift in your attention, to hold you there where you feel discomfort, where the edges soften gradually to ease the blow. Holding is not the same as anaesthetizing and fantasy is not the same as real life. I write because it stops me from cutting but then, softly and quietly, the text bleeds as well. How much of pain is authorized, nurtured, nourished, numbed by the spaces of ordinary living? How much of it can be interrupted or dissolved by the imagining and seeking of alternatives? I am bound to the everyday. I live and breathe its promise. But my attachment to this life is resulting in my own slow death. I want to be jarred, to be forced into desiring and become disorganized, on top of all that. I want to bleed, to eat, to lick, to starve, to think, to do, to retch, to break, to burn, to fade and I want theory—*I want writing*—to let me in on the secret and to tell me why I want it. Can a theory of self-harm contain or engender a theory of sex/sexuality?

The Erotics of Knowing

There are some things, and some people, I think I know only in writing. In the years since Eve Sedgwick's death there has been a stunning outpouring of scholarship, remembrances, tributes, and testaments, all of which speaks not only to the formative role she played in the shaping of queer studies but also to who she was and what she meant to people as a writer, a theorist, a critic, a teacher, a friend, and a mentor. Her death has seen the creation of various panels, symposiums, websites, books, articles, special issues of academic journals, as people from different walks of life—activist, artist, spiritualist, scholar—have sought to celebrate and honour her memory.

Among those who consider themselves her people there has been debate and dialogue—convivial, intense, energetic and alive; all of it has had the effect of holding her ideas close and keeping the buzz going. After her death, many of us still want to be with Eve. We want to meet her again in her texts, to feel the reverberation of her high-pitched laughter, to be surprised and embarrassed anew by the boldness and generosity with which she invited us to open ourselves up to the wide range of possibilities condensed in the notion of sexual identity and to inject the academy, finally, with a good, hefty dose of the erotic.

Theory's Queer Desire/ A Desire for Queer Theory

I was in my mid twenties when I first met Sedgwick. It was a purely textual encounter (all of our meetings were) but the force of it, the way that it got hold of me and made me think and feel so hard was something I had not experienced up to that point. I did not anticipate it happening and yet once it did, it was, decidedly, the thing I wanted. The kind of thinking I did in my first readings of *Epistemology of the Closet* and *Tendencies* felt *good*: it was raw, sharp, piercing. There were edges to it, jutting and jagged. Conceptually, I was approaching this work with intensity and yearning similar only to that with which I engaged life at a physiological or bodily level. Starved, it was as if I was walking around and around and around a set of problems, burning every last ounce of energy to get inside them, to know their contents, to scrape them smooth, to change their contours. On the one hand, I was exhausting myself and wearing myself out from wanting to be crushed so completely by ideas, and on the other, from being absorbed by a crush that everyday kept me charged, exhilarated, anxious, mad with feeling.

Before I happened upon Sedgwick and became absorbed in her work, I used to think about theory as a kind of refuge, a space that I could escape to, that could hold or contain feeling or help create distance from it. I imagined, despite evidence to the contrary, that theory was a bit like the classroom: a mostly safe and innocuous space where nothing too exciting happened, where feeling and emotion were muted, where the primary things that circulated were words and ideas, and maybe, less frequently, provocations to stop and pay attention. I couldn't tolerate the thought of either theory or the classroom as spaces for love and desire.

In my personal life, I could not close the door on anxiety, and while I dreamed that I would die from a specific strain of feeling or desire that had no recognized form to hold it, I wished in my intellectual life that a space could be opened up and filled with countless characterless objects. I wanted things spread out but enclosed. I wanted to lie with someone intimately but be familiar with their shape rather than their smell, to remember their eyes—not their expression but their colour—hazel, brown, or maybe dark blue. Before reading Sedgwick, I had very little idea that masochism could be a distinctly mental matter or that the verbal could be the scene within which my fantasies played out. I had a notion but few resources ultimately for apprehending how learning could feel like lust, or how robustly ideas could attach to people, or how and why I could want a professor to want me when the gift of her knowledge and praise was such teasing—a lavishing before a swift and brutal withdrawal. All of this desiring involved bodies and yet physicality, I was to learn from Sedgwick, wasn't the half of it.

Of the many lasting and profound contributions Sedgwick's theorizing has made to the field of queer studies, it is the rethinking and broadening of the term "sex" to include an "array of acts, expectations, narratives, pleasures, identity-formations, and knowledges, in both women and men, that tends to cluster most densely around certain genital sensations but is not adequately defined by them" that is arguably the most moving and deeply disorienting (1990, p. 29). Defined in this way, Sedgwick's notion of sex, though it resonates perhaps with some of our most basic concepts, differs quite substantially in that it does not presume that sex is a predominantly singular or easily identifiable, knowable thing. Among scholars of queer theory it has prompted renewed and careful reconsideration of queer as an identity category and so has led Elizabeth Freeman, for example, to ask: "Wasn't my being queer, in the first instance, about finding sex where it was not supposed to be, failing to find it where it was, finding that sex was not, after all, what I thought it was?" (2011, p. 32).

Cheeky and brilliant and resplendent as she was, Sedgwick often stated that one of her main ambitions as a writer and a teacher was to make her readers and students "smarter." It is difficult to know what she meant by that or how she imagined that transformation might be measured and tracked. Certainly, the ambiguity of the definitions she provided could not have helped many of us to *feel* much smarter since a characteristic effect of her work in this regard was that of weakening our hold of the things we thought we knew and the axioms by which we lived. And yet, it does seem significant that the intellectual referent of the word "smart" derives, as Lauren Berlant has astutely observed, "from its root in physical pain" (2002, p. 87). This was Eve's S/M paradigm: whether in theory or pedagogy she was compelled to whip us intellectually into shape. As her readers and students we needed to be desirous and willing.

Sex and Reparation

I think that many people (and I am among them) are trying, in our work and in our day to day, using some variant of the notion of queer performativity that Sedgwick bequeathed to us perhaps, to make reparations to the single, most deeply fraught part of our subjectivity: our sexuality. In Sedgwick's terms, queer is a "speech act" that is a provisional and inherently unstable declaration that brings something about rather than simply describing something that already exists. Part of the work of queer performativity, she says, is to exhibit fantasies otherwise experienced as shameful. A "strategy for the production of meaning and being, in relation to the affect of shame," it is motivated by the desire to performatively reconstitute the "interpersonal bridge" that is thwarted when we fail to elicit another's positive interest, and to quell our humiliation without denying the experience of shame (2003, p. 61). Therefore, as a kind of exhibitionism, it is not reductively narcissistic. It exemplifies the ethic that Michael Warner defines as the basis for queer "sociability," specifically the "acknowledgment of all that is most abject and least reputable in oneself" (1999, p. 35).

It feels scary to say that what is "abject" in me, though I imagine Sedgwick might be genuinely interested to know, is the edginess, intense self-destructiveness, and deep down delirious longing that permeates the space of my sexuality and makes the experience of sex seem like my own undoing. In solidarity with Sedgwick as she painfully recollects scenes from her childhood to her therapist while trying to think about her "precocity, its queerness, its sinister ramifications," I am besieged by bitterness at my own "problem" body and the early growth spurt that made me feel like a freakish giant, too tall and heavy and fat, too "sexual," really, to be considered a child by many of the adults around me (p. 30). I can recall at a young age how I hungered for everything and was ravaged by desire and appetite, whether for material things, or love and affection—a cool, caressing touch on my burning hot flesh.

Whatever shape or form it took, I was aware that wanting was a bad and frightening thing, that lacking models for it, permission to act on it, and a sense that my own desires were valid and good and satiable, I needed to transform it, drive it underground, channel it into a safer place. Starving, in its inimitably perverse way and in exaggerated form, thus, capitulated to a wide array of feelings (some inherited from my family, most of them supported by culture) about female desires and bodies, to the idea that there is something inherently shameful and flawed about the female form, something that requires vigilant monitoring and control.

As an anorexic, I rule my appetite with an unbending will. My body is taut and bolted down. My despair and dissatisfaction are etched as if with a scalpel, firm and deep into my skin. Pain and torment centrally define my illness and yet there is something more: it is a feeling, a frantic, buzzing hum and an all-consuming energy. It is pride twisted with power shot through with masochistic pleasure. In a way that queerly and uncannily echoes Sedgwick's description of masturbating as a "holding environment" (p. 165), a space to manage anxieties, and to escape the sometimes cruel experience of family life, it is, for me, "what feels like sex … something that I [can] yearn toward and be lost in the atmosphere of. To me, a whole world." (pp. 165, 45).

Starving for Feeling

When I think about what it feels like to starve, I imagine that there are few things that feel more like flourishing, few things that *can ever feel* as intense—or charged or magnetic—as the deep pressing throb of physical hunger and the stomach pulling tight and inward, inward, inward. In a second I can summon it, that hunger that was like air to me, that ache that was my body's pulse. In recovery, I spent years trying to find strategies to cope with it, to get over it and forget it, and to practice other ways of being that didn't require physical suffering as the single most salient piece of evidence that a life was being lived. That I grieved profoundly the loss of my anorexia and was overcome with feelings of loneliness, emptiness, and yearning for the thing that I had given up and that I imagined was as protective and deeply reliable as my closest friend, was just proof, I guess, of how hard I'd fallen for it, how completely and helplessly I'd been penetrated by my desire.

Anorexia wasn't my first crush, but it has been my most fervent and enduring one. If today I can't have it because for complicated reasons, and a deep-seated fear of disappointing and being shamed by others I've promised to be "good," then I am still no less enthralled by the thought of it. I am still enslaved by the force it exerts in my life and how intoxicating it feels to so determinedly refuse the thing that nurtures me and that I want and need the most. I am envious when I see the signs of it in another. As much as I desire to be bound to it, I want even more to experience (again) the feeling of being bound *by* it: how it simultaneously holds and defeats me, enraptures and destroys me. Daily, I covet it, flirt with it, court it, and solicit it. I want it and I am willing. Writing is like issuing an invitation to it—or not—since I am completely at its mercy. I have no will to speak of when I am in its presence. Its visitation is my absolute surrender. Still.

Thinking—Feeling—Desiring

There is something so devastatingly hot about intellect, particularly one that deals in the queer relational modes of permeability and promiscuity, that performs knowledge as a vastly spacious, improvisatory, and circuitous field, and holds open the possibility of being crushed by and reciprocating desire for what seem the unlikeliest thoughts, things, and people. I am thinking about the ways in which Sedgwick conceived of the word "queer," how as a theoretical tool she imagined it helped make the field of sexuality bigger, more expansive and inviting, so that culture at large could be seen as underwritten by sexual desire, and how it named all the things that cannot be made to signify "monolithically," spaces where "*everything does not mean the same thing*!" (1993, p. 6). I am listening in my mind to Sedgwick articulate the spaces of open possibility and contradiction *within* queerness, observing that one of the most exciting things about it is that it needn't just be about sexuality; it can be about different things, too. I am taking in the various scenes within which, ever concerned with the performative, she eagerly and cleverly spins "queer" outward, along different axes of meaning, exploring how it references and also enacts a certain unsettling in relation to heteronormativity, and marvelling at how the most wonderfully demonstrative aspect of the whole exercise is, ultimately, and unpredictably, the one that turns inward and is self-referential. She writes:

> It's funny, in spite of how homely-looking I am and how shy, I think a fair number of people think of me as even an unusually sexy person. And it's not a facade, at all. The thinking, writing, talking, all the sociality and the political struggle around sex: those are the most vibrant things in my life. It's just they don't connect up genitally for me...at all. (1999, p. 44)

It is the shocking realization that studying and thinking intimately with someone can thoroughly dislocate your habitual relation to cognition and forms of mastery and undermine the truths you have taken to be self-evident. That it can have the effect of making you feel that you've been mastered and brought ecstatically to your knees. Influence is too ordinary a word to describe the hold Sedgwick had on people. It unproductively explains why, eleven years after her death, we are still submitting as boldly and willingly as we ever did, despite the anxiety it can bring, to her experimental, erotic tutelage in unknowing. She was steadfast in her efforts to think differently, and to that end she successfully organized against "the name of the familiar" as a structure of knowing that upholds the value of what seems abjectly and intolerably tied to sameness. Unconvinced that knowledge was something to be gained and prescribed, she was interested instead in thinking about the performativity of knowledge or what the pursuit and production of knowledge *does*. She was attentive in much of her work to the difference that obtains between knowing something and realizing something and although she understood this distinction to be a "densely processual undertaking that can require years or lifetimes," she was notably impelled in her own process by a cancer diagnosis and an encounter with possible death (2003, p. 167).

For Sedgwick, the crisis incurred by illness was an epistemological one. What paralyzed her was not the reality of being sick, having to undergo surgery, or dealing with the likelihood of death, but the narrow ways of thinking illness compels us to adopt. At the beginning of *A Dialogue on Love* she describes her 50/50 percent survival chance as "perfect for turning this particular person inside-out" (1999, p.5). She is clear that it is not what lies at either side of the slash mark that disturbs her; rather, the either-or quality of this dualism *itself* divides her from the world. The challenge in her autobiographical illness narrative then reveals a reparative motive: to use writing to revitalize an epistemological framework depending on multiplicity in the face of cancer's crude oppositions. What accomplishes this task is the discovery of a queer genre that can accommodate all her complexity and open up a space big enough to hold and develop her theories of intersubjective relation and thematic multiplicity.

Commenting that "what I wanted to make palpable—and available—was the quality of a specific listening space, a space that is open to every anxiety but resists propelling onward its fatal itinerary," Sedgwick adopts an ancient Japanese poetic form called *haibun*, which mixes prose with haiku (2006, p. 6). When she weaves haiku into her prose the white space between lines, between poetry and prose become the empty spaces through which many meanings pass. This is, for Sedgwick, reparation writ large: the use of a multiplicity of perspectives to replace dualistic thinking with a more open epistemology, and the writing of a text that, in privileging processes and practices of realization and understanding, prompts other ways of thinking about illness.

* * *

It will be eight years next month since I received, for the third time in my life, the medical diagnosis of anorexia nervosa and entered into treatment. And yet, despite my commitment to my program and the continual effort I've made to build a more sustaining definition of well-being, I am still not very "well," not nearly "recovered." Perhaps it has something to do with the complexity of the illness, by which I mean that, far from manifesting as a random response to trauma or bespeaking a silly narcissism, such as the desire to drop some pounds or to have the "perfect" body, it is in fact a very real and dangerous mental illness, a chronic condition that results in death for about twenty percent of sufferers, either from medical complications or suicide. Sedgwick writes about her depression, that "I thought I'd know when therapy was successful because I'd stop feeling the want of being dead" (2006, p. 8). Even now, along with her, I feel the ache of that want and know it intimately. I am endlessly figuring out ways (on good days) to endure, rather than succumb to its pull. That is to say nothing of the bad days, however, when an obliterating numbness prevails. I am so fucking scared of not feeling. I starve and self-punish to hurt. The throbbing, relentless emptiness; the sharp, frenzied buzz of hunger; the fierce, anxious, anguished work of refusal: all of it lets me know I am still in my body, still breathing and alive.

To the extent that I not only value as an important conceptual tool but also hold close, having adopted it as a mantra for how to live, one of the most elegant and potentially restorative arguments Sedgwick ever proffered, the deceptively simple: "People are different from each other" (1990, p. 23), I can remain open to the possibility that the lure of self-starvation for *some* people is its overwhelming deadening effect. One does not need to suffer from or even know very much about anorexia to have a sense of the degree to which the *visibility* of the anorexic body makes it particularly accessible and susceptible to being overwritten in certain ways. It is the anorexic body that immediately shocks the observer; it is the anorexic body that is frequently the focus of media controversy and intrigue; it is the anorexic body that is rendered by medical and psychiatric knowledges alike as staging a silent but spectacular protest against the inevitable fact of developing into "adult femaleness."

Against this view of the body as strictly surface-sign, however, I wish to point out that the either/or thinking which pervades western culture—positing anorexia as an individual pathology triggered by "cultural forces" that are mostly external to the psyche—has the real consequence of completely eclipsing the experience of the self. For a long time now and particularly since my dissertation, I've been wading knee-deep through reams of theoretical literature, struggling to find a space therein which recognizes anorexia's specificity as an embodied subjectivity, not only as it is represented but *as it is felt*. My preoccupation with endeavouring to think about and also put into words and describe the reality of *being* anorexic in a way that can get close to the heart of what it *feels* like develops from my own stubborn sense that something important is missing in the medical and critical cultural discourses which privilege the visual as a way of knowing.

In my experience, the desire to be thin does not nearly explain the addictive aspect of self-starvation, the constant and compulsive self-denial, and the habitual seeking of death.

Neither does it begin to account for the significance of anorexia as a form of self-knowledge, the meanings of hunger as a perpetual mode of being, and the kinds of refusals it performs. I want to know and have a vocabulary to be able to talk about and interpret *what the hunger means*. I want to develop a form of writing and find a genre that can be open and spacious and experimental enough to explore the affective and sentient aspects of anorexic embodiment as distinctly and seductively queer. I want people to know and not feel shame that intoxicating and perverse pleasure also defines anorexic experience, that it is, for this reason, impossible for some of us to separate out our queer and anorexic selves, and that self-inflicted hunger—something ostensibly not at all "like" sex, can be and sometimes is, experienced by some of us *as* sex.

I want *so much* and I even have, as Sedgwick might say, "a motive," and yet it is undoubtedly my depression that at times immobilizes me, keeps me tied to the knowledge that the world is so painfully inadequate to what I need from it (1993, p. 3). Still, writing, Sedgwick reminds us, is a practice for making reparation and finding pleasure and nourishment in our work. One can only dwell in despair for so long before coming around to hope; one must arrive at a place of bad feeling first to learn how destructiveness can be a condition for love. More than just a critical mode, Sedgwick's queer theory of reparation is also a critical life skill. In a way that never fails to address me personally yet makes room for countless others, it serves as a reminder, endlessly and expansively gesturing to the multiple possible ways I can continue to survive.

References

Berlant, Lauren. 2002. Two Girls, Fat and Thin. In *Regarding Sedgwick: Essays on Queer Culture and Critical Theory*, ed. Stephen Barber and David Clark, 71–108. New York: Routledge.

Britzman, Deborah. 2003. *After-Education: Anna Freud, Melanie Klein, and Psychoanalytic Histories of Learning*. Albany: State University of New York.

Cooper, Julia. 2017. *The Last Word: Reviving the Dying Art of Eulogy*. Toronto: Coach House Books.

Freeman, Elizabeth. 2011. Still After. In *After Sex? On Writing Since Queer Theory*, ed. Janet Halley and Andrew Parker, 27–33. Durham: Duke University Press.

Hanson, Eli. 2011. The Future's Eve: Reparative Reading After Sedgwick. *South Atlantic Quarterly* 110(1): 101–119.

Jagose, Annamarie. 2010. Thinkiest. *Australian Humanities Review* 48: 378–381.

Love, Heather. 2010. Truth and Consequences: On Paranoid Reading and Reparative Reading. *Criticism* 52(2): 235–241.

Resilience. (n.d.). In Cambridge English Dictionary.org. Retrieved from https://dictionary.cambridge.org/dictionary/english/resilience.

Sedgwick, Eve Kosofsky. 1990. *Epistemology of the Closet*. Berkeley: University of California Press.

________. 1993. *Tendencies*. London: Routledge.

________. 1999. *A Dialogue on Love*. Boston: Beacon Press.

________. 2003. Paranoid Reading, Reparative Reading; or You're So Paranoid You Probably Think This Introduction is About You. In *Touching Feeling: Affect, Pedagogy, Performativity*. Durham, NC: Duke University Press.

________. 2006. Teaching/Depression. *The Scholar and Feminist Online*, 4(2): 1–12.

Warner, Michael. 1999. *The Trouble With Normal: Sex, Politics, and the Ethics of Queer Life*. Cambridge, MA: Harvard University Press.

CHAPTER 7

"Titled Things": Materiality and Reification in Antidepressant Narratives

Marie Allitt

In her exploration of the history of psychopharmaceuticals, *Blue Dreams* (2018), Lauren Slater discusses the significance of the names of medications. In their earliest form, antidepressants had the preferred term "psychic energizers," which, Slater suggests, "has a whiff of magic to it. It feels more closely allied to a vitamin than to a drug. It calls to mind the ephemeral, immeasurable psyche, with a little fizz now added, as opposed to the plodding and stern term 'antidepressant'" (pp. 144–145). Slater imagines what would have happened if this name had stuck instead: "Would we have been as quick to pathologize depression if the pills to treat it didn't suggest sickness? A psychic energizer is Everyman's medication, while an antidepressant seems destined for the sickest of souls" (p. 145).

While the impacts of the naming of illness are much discussed, Slater demonstrates that naming of cure is equally significant, as both the name

M. Allitt (✉)
University of Oxford, Oxford, England
e-mail: marie.allitt@theology.ox.ac.uk

J. Hollenbach and R. A. McDonald (eds.), *Re/Imagining Depression*,
https://doi.org/10.1007/978-3-030-80554-8_7

and the fundamental materiality of that cure directly influence the individual's experience of ingesting medication. In this chapter, I consider experiences of consuming antidepressants, focusing on three first-hand narratives: Lauren Slater's *Prozac Diary* (1998), and *Blue Dreams* (2018), and Elizabeth Wurtzel's *Prozac Nation* (1994), which all pay particular attention to the relationship between their medication and illness. I term such texts "antidepressant narratives" to emphasize how these pathographies are explicitly shaped by the prescription and consumption of antidepressant medications. This is not an analysis of the efficacy of psychotropics, as every individual and their ill-health are different and the experiences while being on medication vary. Rather, my aim here is to explore and answer, in part, Slater's own question: "Much has been said about the meanings we make of illness, but what about the meanings we make out of cure?" (1998, p. 9). More specifically, I explore the meanings we make of the processes and pragmatics of cure, and the balance between concepts of wellness and illness as they relate to consuming medication.

As long as there have been minds to alter, substances have been made to alter the mind. Over time this has shifted from temporary mood alteration to mood regulation, and has become a vital component of people's lives in the West. Arguably, it was not until regulated prescriptions and the rapid growth of the pharmaceutical industry from the mid-twentieth century onwards, that drugs, specifically pills, have become a part of everyday life (Bennett 2019). In part because of their ubiquity and because "psychotropic pills ... have increasingly come to be those rare nondescript objects which have the most far-reaching impact," very little attention has been given to the lived experience of ingesting medication (Bennett 2019, p. 5). Here, I focus specifically on antidepressants, but there is certainly overlap with other psychotropic medications, for example tranquilizers, such as Valium, and psychostimulants, such as Adderall or Ritalin. I explore the relationship between an individual and the material of their everyday medication, how a person experiences the taking of their medication, and how it affects their life.

The relationship an individual has with their medication can often be turbulent. In the case of depression, there is an embedded hesitancy in choosing to or not to take the antidepressant, which David A. Karp characterizes as "an awkward dance" (2006, p. 7). There is a tension in the moment of taking the tablet: even for someone who has been taking the drug for a number of years, it is a daily choice (or at least a daily responsibility) to ingest it. With each ingestion there is a giving over of the mind to something material, a surrendering of abstract thought to the physical drug.

The significance and power that one little pill can have has exponentially increased from the 1950s onward: from the contraceptive pill, to antidepressants, and everything in between. In a 2003 *Rolling Stone* article, recounting the history of prescription drugs, Elizabeth Wurtzel offers a biting critique of the invention of an industry designed to prey upon the vulnerabilities of ordinary people: "the answer to all your problems in tablet, capsule or gel-cap form," in many ways epitomizing the popular, cultural discourse of prescription medications (2003, p. 103). The increased medicalization of the mind and mood has inevitably coincided with an increase in misinformation from the media and advertising, especially pertaining to their efficacy, over-prescription, and risk, perpetuating an ingrained stigma and assumption surrounding the taking of medication, especially with regards to antidepressant use. Misinformation and negative didacticism are unhelpful at best and harmful at worst, with such discourse affecting who and how people seek treatment and consequently, their personal relationship with medication. Even an individual who has chosen to take medication, even one who has felt the long-term effects (both positive and negative), will still find a struggle between taking and not taking antidepressants, which is ultimately a struggle between who they are while on the medication, and who they are without it.

As the titles of these memoirs suggest, these narratives focus on the drug fluoxetine (better known by its brand name Prozac). It is a drug whose resonance and significance has infiltrated many aspects of society, becoming ubiquitous even to those who have no medical knowledge of or personal connections to it. Prozac has indeed become a character of its own, although whether it can be regarded as a "literary character" is a different line of thought (Metzl 2002, p. 352; Stepnisky 2007, p. 25). In many ways Prozac is metonymic of antidepressants, so the issues raised in this discussion could well apply to any antidepressant drug. The experiences of depression and antidepressant medication described in these memoirs take place in the United States, and so illustrate a specific reality of psychotropic access and use; experiences of depression and antidepressant medication will inevitably vary depending on location, and different national and global healthcare systems. This discussion seeks to diverge from existing discourse around antidepressant use, which maintains the political and social critique of the "popular frenzy" of psychotropic medications (Metzl 2002, p. 349). My discussion here does not ignore these issues, but it does aim to break from the circularity of such conversations to instead focus on the relationship between patient and prescription.

Naming into Existence

Just as there is no quick fix for depression, there is no quick diagnosis. There is no test through which to measure one's mood and biochemical landscape: "There isn't some blood test, akin to those for mononucleosis or HIV, that you can take to find a mental imbalance. And the anecdotal evidence leads only to a lot of chicken-and-egg types of questions" (Wurtzel 1994, p. 306). In a time of increasing desire for quick and unambiguous answers, it is frustrating to not have an immediate diagnosis that points, simply and directly, to a cure. These frustrations are intensified by incomplete knowledge of depression. For example, framing depression as a result of biochemical imbalance is an incomplete story, overlooking not only environmental factors and context, but the patient as a person with a unique history and individual narrative. The obscurity of the biochemical model still dominates, compounded by various diverging opinions among neuroscientists and psychiatrists (Harrington 2019). This untidy and obscure differentiation can take its toll on the patient, affecting how they go about seeking a cure and recovery. In her essay memoir "Black Swans," (1996) Slater explains:

> I had come to think, through my reading and the words of doctors, and especially through my brain's rapid response to a drug, that whatever was wrong with me had a simplistic chemical cause. Such a belief can be devastating to sick people, for on top of their illness they must struggle with the sense that illness lacks any creative possibilities. (p. 43)

The implication that there is "a simplistic chemical cause" infers that there must therefore be a simple chemical cure, which is "so common in today's high tech biomedical era where the focus is relentlessly reductionistic" (Slater 1996, p. 43). Slater illuminates the conflicts in how we see depression, when the culture surrounding its diagnosis and treatment is complicated by the disconnect between psychology and biology.

Wurtzel comes to the same conclusion that the biochemical model is insufficient: "I have gone from a thorough certainty that its origins are in bad biology to a more flexible belief that after an accumulation of life events made my head such an ugly thing to be stuck in, my brain's chemicals started to agree" (1994, p. 306). There is more to the cause of depression, showing us that such a narrow view is isolating and destructive, and that "too often treatments address only half the problem: they focus only on the presence or only on the absence" (Solomon, 2001, p. 19). Perhaps it is no surprise, given the wealth of economic possibilities, that even after all these years and research, doubt endures. Generally speaking, those who have experienced depression first-hand must realize that recovery, cure, or management of depression requires acknowledgement of all factors: it has no immediate test, nor an immediate cure.

If there is a material basis to depression, why do we fail to consider the *material* factors of medication? If we recognize, as Jeffrey N. Stepinsky purports, that "in place of relationships between analyst and the analysed, or even psychiatrist and client, the biomedical era witnesses the growing importance of relationships between individuals and psychiatric technologies" (2007, p. 25), then why is so little attention given to how consumers experience and relate to those psychiatric technologies, specifically psychopharmaceuticals? Jonathan M. Metzl has advanced this kind of focus with *Prozac on the Couch* (2003) offering a history of contemporary American psychiatry which explores "the possibility that psychotropic medications accrue meanings in both medical and popular cultures, meanings that then come back to inform clinical practice" (p. 6). The recent work of Robert Bennett has also developed the relationship between pharmacology and illness in literary, televisual, and filmic narratives, with particular focus on the cultural significance of pills.

Certainly the "first wave" of critical medical humanities, especially a literary critical emphasis on memoir, has successfully foregrounded the patient voice and provoked significant focus on experiences of mental health, but part of the future of the field must attend to "non-human objects and presences," and partake in the "material turn ... which has reoriented the traditional focus of the humanities on culture, mind and language towards an emphasis on nature, bodies and things" (Whitehead and Woods 2016, p. 2, 14). As such, we must consider the role of medication, cure, treatment in terms of its sensory, somatic, and physiological effect entangled with its symbolism. It is this aspect with which I engage here, by addressing the experiential dimensions of antidepressant medication, through a focus on how images of materiality and corporeality reify mental illness, and illuminate and communicate its invisibility.

Absence and Metaphor

So much about mental illness concerns invisibility and absence. The lack of outward physiological symptoms means mental illness is difficult to diagnose, quantify, and treat. However, when we consider contemporary treatments for mental illness, we must not forget early ideas concerning the visualisation of madness, and how significant such histories are to our understandings of mental health and its varied treatment. In the late eighteenth century, throughout the nineteenth and into the early twentieth century, "it was commonplace that forms of insanity, such as melancholy, could be identified by the physical appearance of the person afflicted" with physiognomy, physical descriptions, illustrations, and later photography, used as vital resources in diagnosis and the construction of medical knowledge (Gilman 1988, p. 26). Expression, pose, and manner were all regarded as indicators of the internal, mental state, and contributed to psychiatric discourses (Gilman 1988; Didi-Huberman 2003; Rawling 2017). Despite the presence of a visual discourse for madness, we furthermore must recognise that such ideas are constructed by clinicians, and do not account for the patient experience. A focus on contemporary patient narratives then reveals that there continues to be frustration with the tangibility and visibility of depression.

To combat this, those suffering often reach for metaphors and analogies of tangible substance. William Styron's *Darkness Visible* (2004), for example, identifies such feelings as "indescribable," before employing an extended metaphor of depression as a storm, and returns again and again to "darkness" as the closest indicator (p. 14). In *The Noonday Demon* (2001), Andrew Solomon likens depression to rust on iron, weathering it towards collapse, and offers "A sequence of metaphors –vines, trees, cliffs" (p. 17, 29). For Solomon, metaphor "is the only way to talk about the experience. It's not an easy diagnosis because it depends on metaphors, and the metaphors one patient chooses are different from those selected by another patient" (p. 29). In narrative terms, offering metaphors with an increasing material and concrete focus helps make depression and its symptoms visible.

Not only are there few outward diagnostic markers, and deficiencies in the language with which to communicate it, the experience of depression is typified by gaps and what is missing: "Depression is in an altogether different zone because it involves a complete absence: absence of affect, absence of feeling, absence of response, absence of interest" (Wurtzel 1994, p. 19). One of the defining images of depression is that of incompleteness, which Slater also addresses, "I was incomplete, apparently, without the pill that was, among other things, a plug to stopper some hole in my soul. Perhaps the hole came from a neuronal glitch, the chemical equivalent of a dropped stitch in the knitted yarn of my brain" (1998, pp. 8–9). As Slater's analogy implies, when discussing the most precise chemical and biological processes, the language of metaphor, "a dropped stitch," is immediately needed in order to make the abstract more palpable. Moving into metaphor can tidy up the narrative, filling in the gaps or clarifying in order to reveal the truth of the experience, as Solomon notes, "[m]aybe what is present usurps what becomes absent, and maybe the absence of obfuscatory things reveals what is present" (2001, p. 19).

Throughout these narratives, the mind becomes matter through the pervasive metaphors of the brain as fabric. It is swaddled and given "wrappings"; the brain is "a knotted, tangled ball of yarn" with "a dropped stitch," and there are "places where the denim is worn so thin the skin shows through" (Wurtzel 1994, p. 45; Slater 1998, pp. 9, 178). By envisaging the brain/mind as fabric, we are able to see the "dropped stitch," appreciate the skin that shows through, and recognize that the experience of depression and the consumption of antidepressants continues to be defined by presences and absences, visibility and invisibility.

Throughout *Prozac Diary*, Slater demonstrates that "mov[ing] into metaphor [was] a significant developmental step" in the experience of recovery and is vital to the communication of her personal experiences (1998, p. 19). In one particular passage, she gives us the image of a blind piano tuner, whose competent work is effective but unseen, "A piano tuner used to come to our house ... The piano never looked any different after he'd worked on it, but when I pressed a C key or the black bar of an F minor, the note sprung out richer, as though chocolate and spices had been added to a flat sound" (p. 23). Such a detail in her life furnishes Slater with a material means to convey the effect of the medication:

> It was as though I'd been visited by a blind piano tuner who had crept into my apartment at night, who had tweaked the ivory bones of my body, the taut strings in my skull, and now, when I pressed on myself, the same notes but with a mellower, fuller sound sprang out.
>
> This is what was different – tempo, tone. Not sight, for everything looked the same. Not smell, for everything smelled the same. Not pitch, for the vibrations of the world were just as they'd always been. To describe the subtle but potent shift caused by Prozac is to tussle with failing words, sensations that seep beyond language. (p. 24).

Invisibility persists in this analogy, but rather than as ignorance, invisibility is here mobilized as a way to acknowledge the "subtle but potent shift."

Making It Real

The language of metaphor reifies what is going on in the mind, making the abstract slightly more concrete. Associating depression with something tangible makes the condition not only more humanized and personal, but also bodily. For Slater, taking the antidepressant returns her to her body, and her body to herself: "Returned, I am then, with each daily dose, with the wash of water to take the pill down, returned I am to my stomach, to my skin, to the fabrics of my past" (1998, p. 200). In the material of the pill, in its ingestion, she returns to the tangibility of her body, where her stomach receives the drug and distributes it throughout her body. It is as if consciousness moves throughout her body with the drug, checking in on parts of the body, flowing inwards and out, protecting, reassuring, confirming that the body still exists. The object presence of the medication re-grounds the body as a part of the condition and the cure.

The return to the body, the very fabric of the self, is central to my argument here, in part because of the subtle yet telling inclusions of somatic descriptions in Slater's memoir. In particular the medical encounters with "The Prozac Doctor" offer up examples of the "gulf" between patient and physician, in which the patient is viewed in the general rather than as a subjective body:

> He had all the right gestures. His knowledge was impeccable. He made eye contact with the subject, meaning me. But still, there was something about the way the Prozac Doctor looked at me, and the very technical way he spoke to me, that made me feel he was viewing me generally – swf,

> long psych history, five hospitalizations for depression and anxiety-related problems, poor medication response in past, now referred as outpatient for sudden emergence of OCD – as opposed to me, viewing me, in my specific skin. (Slater 1998, p. 6)

Crucially, in Slater's experience the return to the body is by no means a reduction to *only* a body. Each part of her body contains its story. Each part has a significance and symbol which goes beyond the biological, and she needs this to be realized:

> My hands: had become a problem. Once they had been conduits for pleasure ... They were the part of me that seemed to have the OCD, tense and seeking, tapping things forty, fifty, sixty times ... From my hands I had learned grief. I had learned how the body can leave you, before you have left it. (Slater 1998, pp. 6–7)

It is notable that Slater does not list negative or melancholic thoughts, feeling, moods; she does not refer to her anxieties and inner turmoil, which contribute to her OCD and impedes her functioning. Instead, she illustrates her ill self, the patient sat across from the doctor, as a physical object, with skin, and hands, with fully embodied senses. She draws attention to the scars on her skin that offer evidence of previous self-harm, which are connected to the less visible, but just as tactile, actions and compulsions of her hands.

This "return" to the physical takes on particular poignancy when read in light of the doctor-patient encounter. As Slater remarks, "Psychopharmacology is the one branch of medicine where there is no need for intimacy; neither knives nor stories are an essential part of its practice" (1998, p. 11). This is fundamentally true; the doctor has no need here to place his hands upon the patient's body, nor does he require medical instruments. In this case (but not all), the doctor is familiar with her story from her medical notes. Yet Slater's concern offers that familiar image of the gulf between the doctor and patient, the patient as object as opposed to subject. This can be further understood with consideration for Martyn Evans' materialist approach within critical medical humanities (2016, p. 344). Evans argues that with the reclamation of the patient voice, medicine has lost sight of the patient's body; he suggests that a material turn, taken seriously, is an important step in re-joining body with voice, in the effort for re-centred personhood. While Slater is frustrated by the lack of contact, it is also frustration of the physical and figurative gulf between patient and caregiver. Slater urgently desires to be seen as a corporeal form, one who feels pain, has blood flowing in her veins, and emotions and feelings in her mind and body. She wants to be helped, but the doctor refuses to take on this desired role:

> I wanted him to touch my hands, not really an odd desire, the laying on of hands a practice as ancient as the Bible itself. The Prozac Doctor was biblical to me. I invited him to take on that role, the role every sick person needs her healer to play – not only technician, but poet, priest, theologian, and friend. I know this was asking a lot, poor man, but few people are as full of need and desire as the patient (p. 7).

The origins of the caregiver figure, mythical and typological, concerns physical connection. Slater illustrates frustration for the invisibility of not only mental illness, but of medical involvement: a frustration which can also be more widespread for invisible illnesses or conditions, such as chronic pain. Reassurance through the tangible and tactile is all but impossible in these contexts.

Ingesting Matters

It could be argued, then, that the presence of the medication allows the invisible to become visible. More than validation, antidepressants serve as a visualisation that enables a reification of the abstract. More certainty can be given when there is a literal pill to swallow.

Once the pills are prescribed, Slater muses upon the significance of ingesting them: "Maybe more than anything else, taking a pill, especially a recently developed psychotropic pill about which researchers have more questions than answers, is always an exercise in the existential, because whatever happens happens to your body alone" (Slater 1998, pp. 10–11). Concern for what is being swallowed impacts the connotations of the antidepressant as an object: "[e]ach time you swallow a pill you are swallowing not only a chemical compound but yourself unmoored; you are swallowing the sea, the drift and the drown. A pill makes the inscrutable Sartre solid, brings to life the haunting solitude of a Munch painting" (p. 11). These images typify a paradox of solidity and uncertainty: the sea encapsulates the contradictions between certainty and instability, where a stormy sea is unpredictable, but is familiar in its tides and waves.

Slater's reference to Sartre and existentialism questions what it is that is made "solid": on the one hand, representing obscure understanding, Sartre stands in as an allegory for the unknown. On the other hand, to suggest that his thought is made "solid" implies certainty through reification. Swallowing the pill is somehow taking in both the known and the unknown.

There is further tension regarding the objective and subjective form of the pill in questioning its status as natural or synthetic: "There it lay, cream and green. Tiny black letters were stamped down its side—DISTA—which sounded to me like an astronomy term, the name of a planet in another galaxy." (p. 8). The pill is initially innocuous, but it is quickly cast as otherworldly and unnatural, reinforcing the conflict between what is natural and what is fabricated. Towards the end of her memoir, Slater explains how.

> Prozac has one of the longest half-lives of any medication available. It takes forty-eight hours to excrete just a portion of its chemical metabolites. Like uranium, Prozac glows underground, in the private darkness of our flesh, in the body's bowel, in the deep tissue of lung, both ominously and beautifully radiant (p. 177).

The image of an element glowing and radiating deep within introduces that discomfort of what is synthetic and what is natural, and in turn asks, what is really going on inside? There is uneasiness for the long-term effects of this synthetic, harmful substance.

The chemical manufacture of the pill is further reinforced and remembered by the way in which Slater chooses to ingest it:

> Every noon I took my pill. Instead of just placing it on my tongue and swallowing with water, I unscrewed the capsule. White powder poured into my hands. I tossed the plastic husk away, cradled the healing talc. I tasted it, a burst of bitterness, a gagging. I took it that way every day, the silky slide of Prozac powder, the harshness in my mouth. (p. 40)

There is a desire to get *inside* the pill, an action which breaks apart the chemistry to explore the inner workings. By taking the tablet in this way, Slater refuses to allow its consumption to become instinctual or commonplace. By opening it up and licking up the powder, she deliberately reminds herself of what is inside, of the material it contains, and in so doing reminds herself of what is at stake by swallowing it. She searches beyond the powder in her palm to what she associates with the pill, musing on the "sphere's interior, where, I sometimes imagine, my whole world might live ... a hospital, a nurse, a horse, a love. A scalpel sharp enough to sever or to stitch" (p. 200).

Yet, this anxiety and reinforcement of the pill as synthetic collides with more positive associations, such as nourishment:

> I picture myself as young, sometimes very young, suckling my pills, which are shaped like tiny teats. I take in my nourishment. Like mother's milk, it builds my strength, facilitates the nerve growth in my brain, so my dendrites sprout longer, my axons curl and clutch at new connections, and the soft spot in my head hardens, and hardens again. (Slater 1998, p. 184)

Significantly it is likened not to food but "mother's milk," the ultimate natural source of nourishment at key early developmental stages. There is the overt sense that the consumption of the pill enables becoming and development, even growth and rewiring, as the explicit neurological terms – "nerve," "dendrites," "axons" – imply the healing or creation of new neural pathways. Ultimately the experience of taking the pill is full of contradictions, stemming from both public discourse and personal associations.

Cosmetic Covering

The tension between visibility and invisibility of depression endures as a discourse. Given the legacy of psychoanalysis and the pervading concepts of repression, suppression, and the unconscious, we soon enter the language of concealment, and not far from ideas of covering, hiding, and veiling. In many ways, the outward signs of recovery, cure, or coping are all cosmetic but they give no proof of what is going on beneath. Personal discourse around depression and healing from mental illness often concerns imagery of masking, sometimes using literal or figurative scars to illustrate how the reality of depression goes deep, and remains long after some of the initial symptoms subside. Slater offers an example of this, referring to her literal scars from self-harm, which develops into a metaphor for persevering and remembering rather than hiding or pretending:

> Once her arms were bandaged. Now they are almost perfect. However, if you look very closely you will see a mesh of small scars all up and down, forearm, shoulder, wrist ... The scars, of which she is now so self-conscious, attest to that, and therefore, she does not like to tan. Scar tissue resists the sun. While the rest of the flesh goes golden, it stays white. It will not be blended. A well-meaning friend once suggested she have cosmetic surgery to erase the marks. The idea upset her. She was surprised that it upset her. But listen. Every day she takes pills whose purpose is to hide her history. She needs some sign, some inscription. Even if no one can see it, the truth is there. (Slater 1998, p. 136)

Initially a series of personal remarks upon her connection to the reality and story of her scars, Slater's description moves into areas concerning stigma, judgement, and most explicitly, concern for what endures. Being faced with the suggestion to alter her skin in order to eradicate the scars becomes a deeply significant moment in her development and self-identification. This is one of the points of tension with regards to a personal experience of depression: what is seen or not seen by others, which we can see as situated within a long historical spectrum of stigma, shame, and sharing of stories of mental health/illness, directly relating back to early psychiatric histories, especially institutional.

In his landmark and controversial study *Listening to Prozac* (1994), Peter Kramer explains his self-coined concept of "cosmetic psychopharmacology" and employs analogies, in fundamentally gendered ways, of antidepressant use with makeovers and cosmetic use. The (often drastic) changes that he witnesses in his patients taking Prozac sees Kramer move into language of surfaces and exteriors, suggesting that the antidepressant smooths out "wrinkles" like "plastic surgery" (p. 12). Slater directly references Kramer's study, and picks up on his language of exteriors, extending it into a more astute comment upon the role and effect of the antidepressant:

> Kramer is unequivocal in his belief that Prozac is the Elizabeth Arden of psychopharmacology, a veritable chemical "makeover", a term that implies trickery and shadow, an artful application of powders and creams to hide unsightly blemishes. In short, makeovers are masks that play with depth and space and dimples. (1998, p. 188)

Slater grasps the incongruous language Kramer uses in such a way that she unearths some significant realities about taking antidepressants. She agrees that by taking an antidepressant she is not the person she was before, or the person she would be without it.

The question of authenticity is ubiquitous in discussions of psychotropic medications (Bennett 2019; Karp 2006). If the medication changes who you are, then we are pushed "to ask which wrappings are real" (Slater 1998, p. 200). These issues arise with regards to Slater's long-term commitment and marriage, wherein she is anxious about presenting an inauthentic self: "She wants him to see through. She wants to be transparent so he may observe the shape of her bones, her uterus, the veins, where liquid rushes, carrying her helixed genes, her haemoglobin, her history of red and titled things" (p. 140). It is noteworthy that this is a third person-narrated interlude in her memoir which acts as a literary form of a mask, allowing her to step back and see herself from the viewpoint of another. The imagery of transparency reveals the desire to be seen in the entirety: as a body, with every atom, sinew, gene working within. To be seen as an individual constituted by a personal "history of red and titled things."

Conclusion

What are the meanings we make out of cure? Slater's life writing, in reflecting on the social, cultural, and scientific constructions of illness and medication, questions the endless and complex ways in which the individual relates to their medication. Slater's use of 'cure' seems intentionally ironic, for she is aware that in reality the depression is not cured, it does not disappear, but is treated, managed, and controlled. She adopts the medical binarism, 'cure,' to remind us that it is not a quick solution, and cannot be likened to a successful course of antibiotics. Consuming antidepressants requires a daily re-engagement with the illness: it is a physical reminder, and quickly a chemical dependence. Slater and Wurtzel's memoirs help demonstrate the complex symbolism, significance, and daily relationship between individual and the antidepressants, which fluctuates between: ambivalence, antagonism, nourishment, stigma, and solution. In order to understand what meaning is made out of 'cure,' out of the use of antidepressants, I suggest that there needs to be specific focus on the lived experience of consumption and ingestion. We cannot sufficiently interrogate notions of identity and selfhood in depression without serious attention to the antidepressants.

Writing within the 1990s and 2000s context of a surge in available pharmaceuticals, and the first generation of antidepressants, Slater and Wurtzel offer just a snapshot into these experiences, which is by no means the whole picture, but rather a starting point. This focus on the materiality of the medication must develop an intersectional focus which directly engages with race, gender, sexuality, class, and geography. Furthermore, it must explore broad representations of pharmaceuticals in a range of media, as Metzl and Bennett have begun to demonstrate in their readings of advertising, film, and television. Genres outside of life writing also provide necessary insight into attitudes of psychotropics: for example, the irony of Ottessa Moshfegh's *My Year of Rest and Relaxation* (2018), parodies the pharmaceutical industry and critiques both US healthcare and contemporary reliance on pharmaceuticals, while simultaneously reaffirming the fully embodied response to antidepressants.

This chapter proposes a distinct focus on the materiality of medication and in turn the effect this has on the patient's identity. How does the pill (physically, culturally) construct the person; the illness; the treatment? Thus far, the materiality of antidepressants has been much overlooked, which has in turn forgotten the body. Might recourse to materiality and material images help us to remember and reconceive of the whole body? Might it further help us stomach the opacity of the biochemical model and the invisibility of depression? It often seems that discourses of depression and readings of depression memoirs are only interested in the brain, but a reorientation to the objects, the bodies, the emotions, recognition for the swallowed pill can tell us more about depression, and in turn reveal so far undisclosed aspects of chronicity, long-term management of symptoms, and treatment for further psychological and physical illnesses.

References

Bennett, Robert. 2019. *Pill*. London and New York: Bloomsbury Academic.

Didi-Huberman, Georges. 2003. *Invention of Hysteria: Charcot and the photographic iconography of the Salpêtrière*. Cambridge, Mass. and London: MIT Press.

Evans, Martyn. 2016. Medical Humanities and The Place of Wonder. In *The Edinburgh Companion to the Critical Medical Humanities*, ed. Anne Whitehead, Angela Woods, Sarah Atkinson, Jane Macnaughton, and Jennifer Richards, 340–353. Edinburgh: Edinburgh University Press.

Gilman, Sander. 1988. *Disease and Representation: Images of Illness from Madness to AIDS*. Ithaca: Cornell University Press.
Harrington, Anne. 2019. *Mind Fixers: Psychiatry's Troubled Search for the Biology of Mental Illness*. London and New York: W.W. Norton & Company.
Karp, David A. 2006. *Is It Me or My Meds?* London and Cambridge, Mass.: Harvard University Press.
Kramer, Peter. 1994. *Listening to Prozac*. London: Fourth Estate.
Metzl, Jonathan M. 2002. Prozac and the Pharmacokinetics of Narrative Form. *Signs* 27 (2): 347–380.
———. 2003. *Prozac on the Couch*. Durham and London: Duke University Press.
Moshfegh, Ottessa. 2019. *2018*. My Year of Rest and Relaxation. London: Vintage.
Rawling, Katherine D. B. 2017. "She sits all day in the attitude depicted in the photo": Photography and the psychiatric patient in the late nineteenth century. *Medical Humanities* 43: 99–110.
Slater, Lauren. 1996. Black Swans. *The Missouri Review* 191: 29–46.
———. 1999. *1998*. Prozac Diary. New York: Penguin Books.
———. 2018. *Blue Dreams: The Science and the Story of the Drugs That Changed Our Minds*. New York: Little, Brown and Company.
Solomon, Andrew. 2001. *The Noonday Demon: An Atlas of Depression*. New York and London: Scribner.
Stepnisky, Jeffrey N. 2007. Narrative Magic and the Construction of Selfhood in Antidepressant Advertising. *Bulletin of Science, Technology & Society* 27 (1): 24–36.
Styron, William. 2004. *1990*. Darkness Visible. London: Vintage.
Whitehead, Anne, and Angela Woods. 2016. Introduction. In *The Edinburgh Companion to the Critical Medical Humanities*, ed. Anne Whitehead, Angela Woods, Sarah Atkinson, Jane Macnaughton, and Jennifer Richards, 2–25. Edinburgh: Edinburgh University Press.
Wurtzel, Elizabeth. 1994. *Prozac Nation: Young and Depressed in America*, 2005. London: Quartet Books Limited.
———. 2003. American Icons: The pill. *Rolling Stone* 922: 103–105.

CHAPTER 8

Variations on Depression in the Work of Ken Lum

Sima Godfrey and Ken Lum

I no longer remember when I first met Ken Lum. Both of us were teaching at the University of British Columbia and somewhere along the way we moved from being colleagues to friends. Sad as I was when he left for Philadelphia, I was convinced this was an important step for him—not just professionally but personally. Vancouver is a city fraught with memories for him—memories of a difficult, disrupted childhood as the son of a Chinese immigrant mother struggling to stay afloat; memories of his time as a depressed chemistry student at Simon Fraser University; happier memories of being a sign painter; memories of starting an MFA at New York University and then rushing back to Vancouver the

The correction of this chapter can be found under https://doi.org/10.1007/978-3-030-80554-8_16

S. Godfrey (✉)
Department of French, Hispanic and Italian Studies, University of British Columbia, Vancouver, BC, Canada
e-mail: sima.godfrey@ubc.ca

K. Lum
University of Pennsylvania, Philadelphia, PA, USA
e-mail: ken.lum@monumentlab.com

J. Hollenbach and R. A. McDonald (eds.), *Re/Imagining Depression*, https://doi.org/10.1007/978-3-030-80554-8_8

following year to attend to his ailing mother; memories of his less than hospitable transfer to the University of British Columbia where his talent was too often resented rather than praised; and, ultimately, memories of his triumphant leap into the Vancouver artworld. He has left an indelible mark on the city with his *Monument to East Vancouver* from 2010 (familiarly known as *The East Van Cross*). But at some point, I believed—and as his honorary Jewish mother I told him so—that Ken had to break away from Vancouver to rethink those experiences and insights from a distance, on a bigger stage. To this day I miss our conversations over lunch.

Despite the title of his well-known *Mirror Maze with 12 Signs of Depression* (2002), I never associated Ken's art with depression, except to the extent that ongoing social inequities based on money, class, race, ethnicity, marginalization or perceived irrelevance produced in him a sense of existential depression.

What I call existential depression in Ken's work coincides with the idea of a "public feeling," such as Ann Cvetkovich has described in her book, *Depression: A Public Feeling*. It is a cultural and social phenomenon. In the spirit of "public feelings" depression, as Cvetkovich characterizes it, describes "the affective dimensions of ordinary life" the investigation of which "emerges from important traditions of describing *how capitalism feels*" (original emphasis, Cvetkovich 2012, p. 11).

That the social inequities of capitalism produce a depressive affect in Ken Lum's work is clear. Without being able to articulate it at the time, however, beyond these kinds of expressions of depression what I intuitively sensed in Ken and his work was what David Eng and Shinee Han in their book, *Dialogue on Racial Melancholia and Racial Dissociation: On the Social and Psychic Lives of Asian Americans* identify as melancholia. Not melancholia in the strictly Freudian sense, but melancholia as "a compelling framework to conceptualize registers of loss and depression attendant to social and psychic processes *of immigration, assimilation, and racialization*" (my emphasis, Eng and Shinhee 2019, p. 35). In Eng and Han's account melancholia does not represent a pathology but functions as "a necessary process of political engagement and action. It is the work of renarrating loss and rebuilding communities" (p. 61). The melancholia they describe offers a productive twist on the existential depression and empathy I felt in Ken's writings and his work and one that ultimately invigorates it with a latent agenda.

At the time of my conversation with Ken in the summer of 2020, however, it was depression, not melancholia, that was on the table.

Sima Godfrey: Is it fair to say that in your work you are less interested in the individual, personal psychological experience of depression than in the existential condition of depression?

Ken Lum: Yes, I'm more interested in the existential condition of depression, as you put it. The connection between actual psychological depression and the individual interests me as a human being but the binary tethering creativity and depression is also something amplified by the art system for a myriad of reasons, including marketing. We like to think of artists as restive or crazy for which if not for art, they would be long dead. There is some truth to this. I became an artist in order to have a life of my choosing, not one imposed upon me.

Godfrey: There is the romantic cliché of the depressed artist that, as you suggest, the art market has often exploited. That is clearly not you. But would it be correct to say that depression inhabits much of your work?

Lum: I have often revisited the idea of depression because I'm interested in the problem of psychic damage at both the individual and societal levels. I have always thought of art as providing me with a way to speak about things that are difficult to announce. Life is full of stress, especially for the poor and vulnerable. I haven't seen the world become less stressful for most people. I have also noticed how few artists deal specifically with this topic because it is not an easy topic to deal with.

I feel that the times have aligned with my work, so as an artist, I am lucky in that sense. I have for a long time been interested in expressing something within the space of what can and cannot be said, of what can and cannot be expressed. I have said as much in many interviews over the years. Well, we are in a moment where we are deeply challenged by language to express the times we are in. It is why the term 'unbelievable' has been bandied about so much, because it is unbelievable and yet we have to believe the reality that swamps us presently. My work is often barely optimistic in the sense that I seek glimmers of subjectivity—cries for help, perhaps—that are all but encased behind the system of commercial signs and other prevalent representational systems. In that sense, the slide from hope to hopelessness or turn from hopelessness to hope is short. It is the reason, I think, why I received so much negative opinion in Canada when I started out. My work was never about redemption, but what was real. It was always concerned with facing up to the real and then asking the question: and then what?

Godfrey: I have hesitated at the idea of depression as generating your work because the emotion I associate with it and with your writing is empathy. Rather than an emotion, I wonder if depression—personal or societal—is an organizing principle for you as it was in your work, *Mirror Maze with 12 Signs of Depression*?

Lum: Depression can be an organizing principle in my work. Why not? Or it can be other terms such as despair, anxiousness, withdrawal, inwardness, and incapacitation. They are all variations on a theme: the psychological and bodily damage exacted on humans (and nature) by the world of organized capital. People crying for help is a recurring subject in my work. Or people at the limits of language. It is not helplessness that I am interested in exploring so much as it is the humanity *in* helplessness. My hope is always the engendering of empathy in the viewer as a starting point for a critique of the way things are. *Mirror Maze with 12 Signs of Depression* is a title that plays with words. The *with* in the title can function connectively, as a preposition connecting two distinct components of the work, that of the mirror maze structure and that of the text features. But it can also function descriptively as in the mirror structure itself is depressed.

Godfrey: So is depression, then, the word you would routinely use to speak about the affect in your work?

Lum: I prefer "despair" to "depression" in describing an ongoing concern in my work. "Despair" is less clinical and more a condition, at least to me. In *Mirror Maze with 12 Signs of Depression*, I was suggesting that the identification of the Self with the mirror produces feelings of depression. To look oneself in the mirror is still used to face up to oneself as though the mirror on its own can furnish that possibility. Depression is the logical mental result for the privileging of the mirror as the paragon of the Self. That is why the work was sited in the enlightenment design of the Orangerie gardens in Kassel, with its radiating concourses of water channels and grass corridors.

Godfrey: How did your first public respond to that work? Were they unsettled?

Lum: The visitor experience was much more disconcerting than I anticipated. There was a real confusion of time and space. A student who was monitoring the exit of the work took it upon himself to poll visitors about the amount of time they thought they spent in the mirror maze. While unscientific, the responses were informative. Visitors thought they spent ten to fifteen minutes in the pavilion when in fact the average amount of time spent was closer to a mere four minutes.

Godfrey: It is easy to see why visitors come out of *Mirror Maze* disoriented by their fractured image. That moment of destabilization could be read as a psychic sign of depression.

On a more formal level, I have always been fascinated by your longstanding interest in signs. Do you see other works of yours functioning as signs of depression? Billboard-type signs, semiotic signs?

Lum: Yes. For instance in my shopkeeper series, the movable or replaceable letters, one half of the works, are cries for help. They express something of the subjectivity of the proprietor of the shop. They are expressions that are at odds with sound business sense—stay away from public pronouncements that can hurt business. The image/repeated text series are configured within the sign system of advertising, but they speak to moments of incapacitation rather than a directive to buy. The works oscillate between image and text rather than point the way to the supermarket or store. The depicted persons are in situations where language is at its limits and fails them. As a result, their respective identities come into question. So much of my works call up commercial signage, the life-sucking symbol par excellence of capitalism. So, yes, you could say the signs are also signs of depression.

Godfrey: For me those signs of depression are also expressions of empathy.

Lum: Perhaps it is my nature or expectation of art but I cannot look at something without thinking about what is excluded or not there. For example, when I look at a publicly sited statue, I think about who has not been publicly acknowledged, and why. I don't just think of the statue that I am beholding but the inventory of statues that dot the civic or wider landscape. My interest in commercial signage is not a Pop Art fascination with upsetting the cart of high art or a cold read of the industrially produced graphics and material surfaces that dominate the visual field, although I am influenced by Pop Art. My interest is in the subjectivities that are palpable and enmeshed *within* the graphics and material surfaces. For example, the community of store owners as expressed in my minimall series, or the proprietors as imagined to exist in my shopkeeper works. Or the imagined deceased in the necrology series. The complexity and fullness of being human is often in a collision course with the suppressing forces of the social economy. The human quality is often barely detectable (as in Pop Art), so contained is the human condition. But I am not interested in expressing some redemptive possibility of escape or transcendence from the world as constructed. I am interested in expressing the struggle to survive this world, not necessarily the struggle to challenge this world or even to reimagine this world anew.

Godfrey: At some level all your work reflects the uneasy relationship between individuals and their shaky place in or exclusion from their socioeconomic context. Currently, during the pandemic, we are dealing with an extraordinary conjunction of personal, private depression, and very public economic depression. How do you see your art responding to or articulating this new environment?

Lum: I see my work aligning and giving expression to the problem of people who struggle just to keep their heads above water. It has been a concern of mine for a very long time. That my work is especially articulating this present moment of pandemic is because the struggle to survive for many has become magnified to an intolerable level. As such, the social tensions explored in my art move commensurately with the real social tensions that are actually taking place. I am very much interested in producing through my art an experience in the viewer of inhabiting the subjectivity of another, albeit one that is imagined but a subjectivity that is plausible to exist. I try to achieve this effect or experience by a formal composition in my art that calls up non-art scenarios. I like to defer the recognition of my art as art such that the viewer is made to think about real life situations, however momentary, before the work's art status is resumed to be recognized.

During this time, I have never been busier. I think it is important to not just continue to work but to work in new ways. I have always done that since as long as I can remember. I think that is the stock and trade of coming from where I came from. I learned to multi-task from a tender age. Not necessarily a good thing as directedness and focus are privileges of a more advantaged background. But during this time, as you know, I was able to revise a screenplay about Chinese contract laborers.

Godfrey: It is exciting to see you confront the challenges of this unsettling new environment in a new medium. When the film gets produced—as I hope it will—it will be a product of the generalized state of depression so many are living through and suffering from. I am certain that it will also be a work of great empathy.

The final aside Ken tossed out at the end of our conversation is telling. Without revealing too much, his film recounts the story of Chinese laborers in pioneer America. It is a narrative of immigration, assimilation and racialization, the kind that Eng and Hee have associated with the psychic splitting of the Asian-American psyche. Eng and Hee add that the melancholia they associate with that splitting is "a mechanism that helps us (re)construct identity and take our dead with us to the various battles we must wage in their names—and in our names" (Eng and Shinhee 2019, p. 43). If I have been impressed with the enormous *empathy* I feel in Ken's work, over and above depression, it is in large part because of his devotion to the battles he wages in the names of the dead, to the losses he narrates. Yes, his work expresses public feelings of despair at crushing social and economic injustice among immigrants and others. It reflects feelings of otherness, exclusion and marginalization. As Ken asserted in our conversation: "I have always thought of art as providing me with a way to speak about things that are difficult to announce. Life is full of stress, especially for the poor and vulnerable." But here I will venture out on a psychic limb with the help of Eng and Hee. Beyond the public feelings of depression his work communicates, as a friend I feel "the things that are difficult to announce," the stress faced by "the poor and vulnerable," represent a private act of homage, most notably to the selfless mother with whom I opened these reflections, a woman who inspired in him more humanity than hopelessness.

References

Cvetkovich, Ann. 2012. *Depression: A Public Feeling*. Durham: Duke University Press.

Eng, David, and Shinhee Han. 2019. *Dialogue on Racial Melancholia and Racial Dissociation: On the Social and Psychic Lives of Asian Americans*. Durham: Duke University Press.

CHAPTER 9

Don't We Hurt Like You? Examining the Lack of Portrayals of African American Women and Mental Health

Nyasha Junior

Hannah Horvath (Lena Dunham) on *Girls* can't stop counting because of her OCD. CIA officer Carrie Mathison (Claire Danes) precariously manages her bipolar disorder on *Homeland*. Toni Collette plays an artist, mother, and wife who must cope with her dissociative identity disorder in *United States of Tara*. Increasingly, we're seeing more women onscreen dealing with mental illness, often in ways that treat their disorder as just one element in a fully human, complex character. But all of these women are white. Women of color—specifically African American women—are not afforded the same type of humanity onscreen, if they're even represented at all.

Originally published in *Bitch Magazine*'s 2015 Summer issue, *Blue*.

N. Junior (✉)
Department of Religion, Temple University, Philadelphia, PA, USA
e-mail: nyasha.junior@temple.edu

J. Hollenbach and R. A. McDonald (eds.), *Re/Imagining Depression*,
https://doi.org/10.1007/978-3-030-80554-8_9

Of the limited shows and films that feature African American women protagonists, only a few have characters with mental illnesses. The lack of images of African American women with mental illness, combined with the myth of the "strong Black woman," contributes to the mistaken notion of mental health issues as "a white-girl thing" and compounds their stigma among African American women. It's no secret that African American women are underrepresented on the big and small screens, especially in starring or lead roles. According to reports from the Center for the Study of Women in Television and Film, among the top-grossing 100 films in 2014, 74% of female characters were Caucasian and 11% were African American. The numbers aren't much different in the realm of television (including cable and Netflix), where 77% of female characters were white and 13% were African American in 2013–2014 (Lauzen 2015, p. 1).

In the infrequent instances when we actually see leading African American women on-screen, their portrayals tend to reinforce the stereotype of the strong Black woman: stoic, hypercompetent superwomen who soldier on without complaint regardless of their circumstances (see Harris 2014). From doting mammy figures to Claire Huxtable to the cool and collected Olivia Pope, these women rarely buckle under pressure, creating the false impression that Black women can (and should) weather any storm. These seemingly positive representations of strength and independence can be damaging, as they discourage African American women from seeing themselves as ordinary women with ordinary struggles.

"It makes people think that the myth of the strong Black woman is something that they really ought to live into," says Chanequa Walker-Barnes, author of the recently published book *Too Heavy a Yoke: Black Women and the Burden of Strength*. "And it makes it much harder [for] people experiencing symptoms of depression to feel that their emotional problems are valid."

* * *

There is limited and somewhat conflicting data on African American women and mental health in part because some studies have small, unrepresentative sample sizes or do not disaggregate data by both race and gender. In "The Epidemiology of Mental Disorders and Mental Health Among African American Women" in *In and Out of Our Right Minds: The Mental Health of African American Women* (2003), Dr. Diane R.

Brown and Dr. Verna M. Keith report that rates of schizophrenia, generalized anxiety disorder, somatization (unexplained physical symptoms of psychological distress), and phobia were highest among African American women (as compared with African American men, white men, and white women). The study found that over the course of a year, almost five African American women out of a hundred were diagnosed with depression. This was similar to the numbers for white women (4.6 out of 100) but much higher than the 1.0 for African American men and 2.1 for white men. Among African American women, the diagnosis of mental disorders is highest for major depression, simple phobia, agoraphobia, social phobia, and PTSD (Brown and Keith 2003).

Lesbian and bisexual women experience higher rates of depression compared with African American women in general, according to a study from UCLA. The National LGBTQ Task Force found that almost half of Black transgender respondents (not separated by gender) have attempted suicide (Grant et al. 2011). These studies highlight how intersections of one's identity may exponentially impact the mental health status of Black women. Some of the risk factors for psychological distress and depressive symptoms among African American women include age, marital status, poverty, poor health, and stressful life events such as financial issues and family conflict. But African American psychologist Dr. Kira Hudson Banks, an assistant professor of psychology at St. Louis University in St. Louis, Missouri, cautions against focusing on particular risk factors. Banks explains, "While it's important to think about the intersection of race, class, and place, there are stressors that you don't escape being a Black woman" (personal communication). She argues that because of discrimination and other factors, even African American women who are affluent and educated face environmental stressors.

Still, Banks cautions against concluding that African American women experience mental illness at inherently higher levels. Instead, she says, "It may be the case that they might be in certain spaces and locations that put them at higher risk for mental health issues." And, although there may be some patterns relating to African American women's risk factors and experiences in the mental health care system, African American women are a complex group and should not be viewed as monolithic. Banks explains, "I try to avoid being too reductionist, too cookie-cutter in discussing Black women's experiences" (personal communication). Banks emphasizes the importance of noting differences among African American women, including socioeconomic status, ethnicity, nationality, sexual identity, and skin tone.

One of the primary barriers to proper diagnosis is the failure of some African American women to recognize symptoms and to realize that they can get help. Walker-Barnes refers to this phenomenon as "walking with broken feet" (Walker-Barnes 2014, p. 43). She coined this phrase to describe the experience of African American women regarding pain not as pathological but as normative. This racialized and gendered "burden of strength" keeps African American women from noticing that something is wrong physically or emotionally because they do not regard it as abnormal. Race, gender, and class affect the particular ways that patients express their psychological distress, and medical professionals who are unaware of these differences may not properly diagnose mental illness among African American women. A lack of cultural competency can also play out in potential misdiagnoses of African American women. Ramou Sarr, cocreator of the podcast *Black Girls Talking* and a freelance writer whose work explores media representations, believes that people who don't readily know many people of color resort to ideas that they learned from television. "They think that that's how Black women are. With such limited [roles] given to Black women, you don't get to see our full range. We aren't given autonomy, and we aren't seen as individuals" (Sarr, personal communication).

This can have dire consequences when it comes to mental health treatment. Despite the prevalence of mental illness among African American women, those who meet the criteria for major depression are often untreated or undertreated as compared with other subgroups. "It would be completely reasonable to suggest that there are Black women who are experiencing depression who are not being identified. One, because they're not accessing the treatment. But two, they might be presenting in a way that looks different than what a clinician is familiar with in terms of depression," Banks says.

Typical symptoms of depression may include depressed mood, anhedonia (loss of pleasure), or lethargy, but African American women do not tend to manifest depression that way. They mask their depression with overactivity, such as being too busy and overscheduling, and report agitation and irritation. They may try to cope through binge eating or compulsive shopping in an effort to self-medicate. According to Banks, research suggests that across races the same set of symptoms will receive different diagnoses (Banks and Kohn-Wood 2002, p. 178). For example, despite presenting with the same symptoms, an African American might be diagnosed with schizophrenia, whereas someone who is white might be diagnosed as bipolar.

Preconceived notions of African American women play out in other ways. "Some clinicians seem to think 'She's a Black woman. She's not crying, so she's fine,' as if Black women don't need mental health services. As if they don't have the ability to break," says Imade Borha, the creator of the blog *Depressed While Black*. She said a psychiatrist refused to prescribe medication to her although she was suicidal. The psychiatrist told her, "You'll be fine; it's just a little phase." For African American women, not presenting in expected ways may mean that they do not receive the same level of care or are not treated with the same urgency as patients of other races. Many African American women recognize that a non-African American therapist might lack understanding and compassion regarding their responsibilities, family expectations, or religious and community obligations. Walker-Barnes says that patients in her practice tell her, "I got tired of having to educate my therapist about my reality" (2014). But finding a culturally competent Black mental health professional creates its own challenge: According to 2014 membership data from the American Psychological Association, only 1.4% of its members self-identified as Black.

Even after recognizing that something might be wrong, the cultural stigma against seeking help is another roadblock in the way of treatment. In their 2004 study, "African Americans' Perceptions of Psychotherapy and Psychotherapists," Vetta L. Sanders Thompson, Anita Bazile, and Maysa Akbar found that cultural and financial barriers, lack of knowledge, and alternative outlets (such as consulting a minister) played a large role in lack of treatment, as well as cultural stigma, which is intertwined with shame and embarrassment. There is an emphasis on the importance of "strength" among African Americans and the desire to resolve family issues internally. Male participants regarded seeking psychotherapy as related to "weakness and diminished pride," while women participants pointed out the "historical requirement that they be the anchor and source of strength in the family."

"It's almost as if the stereotype tells the world Black women are not human," says Borha. "And we don't cry like you. We don't hurt like you. We don't go through pain like you. So we don't need the same level of care—and that's a lie. We need the same level of care that any other human being needs."

* * *

The tide against the recognition of mental health issues is turning thanks to advocacy from Black women offscreen. Chiara de Blasio, daughter of New York City mayor Bill de Blasio, is a mental health advocate and has publicly shared her experiences with substance abuse and depression. She has become a spokesperson for a New York City program aimed at helping young people with depression. Singer Fantasia Barrino, former Destiny's Child member Michelle Williams, and other celebrities have discussed their efforts to cope with depression. First Lady Michelle Obama has helped launch Change Direction, a national effort to educate Americans about mental health issues. These public steps create greater visibility for mental health issues and help dispel the myth that depression does not affect Black women.

As the film and television landscape continues to change, we are slowly seeing more nuanced portrayals of Black women in mainstream pop culture. Borha felt empowered to seek treatment after watching the *Girlfriends* episode where Tracee Ellis Ross's character sees a therapist. "The show made a huge imprint on my life and normalized mental health treatment for Black women." More encouragement comes from the unexpected realm of reality television. For all their staged fights and shallow setups, *Braxton Family Values* and *Real Housewives of Atlanta* have featured several episodes where participants engage in therapy sessions with African American clinical psychologist Dr. Sherry Blake. "Seeing a Black woman as a therapist—that takes some of the mystery and the fear and the stigma out of therapy," says Walker-Barnes (personal communication). While these programs do not really reflect the work involved in long-term therapy—which may scare some people from pursuing counseling—these quick televised consults offer much-needed insight into the process for an audience that is unfamiliar with what therapy can look like. In addition, African American women are creating new communities, spaces, and discourse through YouTube, Tumblr, and web series.

More mainstream depictions are coming, slowly but surely. In the Shonda Rhimes law procedural *How to Get Away with Murder*, Annalise Keating (Viola Davis) is all at once an assertive lawyer, a capable professor, and a person with vulnerabilities. Toward the end of the first season,

Annalise grapples with the investigation of her husband's murder and eventually seeks solace in her mother, Ophelia (Cicely Tyson). Her mother's tough love approach pushes Annalise to a breaking point, and she finally confronts her mother about childhood abuse she endured at the hands of her uncle, Ophelia's brother. Annalise asserts that her husband, a psychology professor, was the only one who truly understood her mental health issues. Ophelia replies, "Ain't no reason to talk about it and get all messy everywhere. Certainly no reason to go to a headshrinker for help and end up marrying him." In a single short scene, viewers are shown both a generational and a cultural gap between Annalise and her mother—for whom the idea of treating one's mental health feels frivolous.

In addition, Andre Lyon (Trai Byers) on the wildly popular *Empire* has bipolar disorder. In her post "Grin and Bear It No More" on the blog *For Harriet*, writer Jordan Maney discusses her struggle and acceptance of her PTSD diagnosis and the impact watching Byers's performance had on her (2015, n.p.). His scenes of "suicidal ideation, the euphoria of mania, the depression that follows, the untethered emotions, the raging thoughts" mirrored her own, perhaps none more significant than "the feeling that to suffer alone and pretend to be fine is better than to speak up and possibly lose everything." She thanked Byers and the show's creators for "bringing reality and humanity to mental health issues seldom explored through the perspective of African Americans on television before."

Television and film portrayals of African American women may seem trivial when compared with such "real world" health issues as poverty and insurance coverage. Still, we consume onscreen images, and they have an effect on our offscreen lives, shaping our understanding of ourselves and others and helping to define our notions of what is normal and expected behavior. In April 2015, Shonda Rhimes was inducted into the National Association of Broadcasters' Broadcasting Hall of Fame. In her acceptance speech, Rhimes said in part, "In Shondaland, our shows look like how the world looks. Everyone can see themselves when they turn on the TV on Thursday nights on ABC. To me, that was not some difficult, brave, special decision I made. It was a human one. Because I am a human." With showrunners like Rhimes, we may be able to see more realistic and honest portrayals of African American women—helping to break down stereotypes and the myth that Black women just don't get blue.

References

Brown, Diane R., and Verna M. Keith. 2003. The Epidemiology of Mental Disorders and Mental Health Among African American Women. In *In and Out of Our Right Minds: The Mental Health of African American Women*, 23–58. New York: Columbia University Press.

Grant, Jaime M., Lisa A. Mottet, Justin Tanis, Jack Harrison, Jody L. Herman, and Mara Keisling. 2011. *Injustice at Every Turn: A Report of the National Transgender Discrimination Survey*. Washington: National Center for Transgender Equality and National Gay and Lesbian Task Force.

Harris, Tamara Winfrey. 2014. Precious Mettle: The Myth of the Strong Black Woman. *Bitchmedia*. https://www.bitchmedia.org/article/precious-mettle-myth-strong-black-woman.

Banks, Kira Hudson, and Laura P. Kohn-Wood. 2002. Gender, Ethnicity and Depression: Intersectionality in Mental Health Research with African American Women. *African American Research PeRspectives* 8 (1): 174–184.

Maney, Jordan. 2015. Grin and Bear It No More: We Need More Honest Media Portrayals of Black Mental Health. *For Harriet*, 14 March. http://www.forharriet.com/2015/03/grin-and-bear-it-no-more-we-need-more.html

Lauzen, Martha M. 2015. It's a Man's (Celluloid) World: On-Screen Representations of Female Characters in the Top 100 Films of 2014. 2014 On-Screen Representations: Report compiled by the Center for the Study of Women in Television and Film, San Diego State University, San Diego, CA. http://womenintvfilm.sdsu.edu/files/2014_Its_a_Mans_World_Report.pdf.

Sarr, Ramou E. 2013. Break Down and Let It All Out: A Study on the Relationship Between the Representation of Black Women. Masters thesis, Harvard University, Boston, MA.

Thompson, V.L.S., A. Bazile, and M. Akbar. 2004. African Americans' Perceptions of Psychotherapy and Psychotherapists. *Professional Psychology: Research and Practice* 35 (1): 19–26.

Walker-Barnes, Chanequa. 2014. *Too Heavy a Yoke: Black Women and the Burden of Strength*. Eugene, OR: Cascade Books.

CHAPTER 10

Feeling Unproductive: Vivek Shraya on the Creative Labor of Negative Affect

Pansee Atta

Vivek Shraya is a multi-talented, multi-disciplinary visual artist, poet, writer, musician, filmmaker, and M.A.C. model. Her novels *The Subtweet* (2020) and *She of the Mountains* (2014) and her non-fiction books *I'm Afraid of Men* (2018) and *Death Threat* (2019, illustrated by Ness Lee) have been published to wide acclaim, as have her far-ranging musical projects, such as the 2017 EP *Part-Time Woman*, which was produced in collaboration with the Queer Songbook Orchestra. Much of her work examines the exigencies of queer, trans, South Asian identity, unreservedly celebrating its pleasures and laying bare its associated pain.

Shraya's practice meditates on the simultaneous pressures of the public desire for—and rejection of—expressions of negative affect by Black, Indigenous, and people of color (BIPOC) artists. In her short film *I want to kill myself* (2017), alongside intimate domestic portraits with her loved ones, Shraya remarks: "I was tormented about how my writing would fail you. (I am not supposed to disclose this because I have a duty as an artist,

The correction of this chapter can be found under https://doi.org/10.1007/978-3-030-80554-8_16

P. Atta (✉)
Carleton University, Ottawa, ON, Canada

J. Hollenbach and R. A. McDonald (eds.), *Re/Imagining Depression*, https://doi.org/10.1007/978-3-030-80554-8_10

as a girl, as a brown person to perform gratefulness)." Speaking the unvarnished truth aloud is framed, however, both as a freedom and a necessity. Shraya concludes:

> Saying *I want to kill myself* made my pain explicit. Saying *I want to kill myself* to the people who love me meant I was shown an immediate and specific kind of care that I desperately needed. Saying *I want to kill myself* kept me alive.

Shraya situates her own experiences of depression and suicidality in a broader socio-political affective context by drawing attention to the failure of individualized manifestations of self-care: "Sometimes no amount of swimming, yoga, eating clean, sleeping, socializing, talking, therapy, leaving town, art making, friendship or love can relieve."

This critique of the sanitized, mass-media representation of depression and trauma is echoed in Shraya's recent photography project *Trauma Clown* (2019), in which she, in costumery reminiscent of a *commedia dell'arte* harlequin, performs an overdramatized display of misery as she is showered with roses on a theatre stage. Drawing attention to the overdetermination of depictions of gendered and racialized trauma, iterations of this image are presented and re-presented in various familiar settings: in a gallery, in a print publication, on a living room wall. Shraya might be understood here as a "vulnerability artist" in José Esteban Muñoz' sense of the term, one that performs vulnerability just as Kafka's "Hunger Artist" performs starvation, taking on an affective burden to elicit an audience's affirmation (Muñoz 2006b, p. 194). Muñoz argues that "the vulnerability artist, like the hunger artist, is undone by her need of affirmative feelings" (p. 199), just as Shraya's *Trauma Clown* participates in the performance of suffering that is symbolically rewarded with roses. But Shraya's performance is a self-reflexive satire of the *labor* of that performance and its consumption by an arts industry that demands its constant re-production under the self-congratulatory guise of a social justice mandate. The roses here stand for more than just emotional affirmation and 'good feelings' (in Sara Ahmed's use of the term); they also carry the real, material implication of continued employment as an artist in a deeply precarious working environment. *Trauma Clown* reminds us that living a queer, racialized life under cis-heteropatriarchal capitalist White supremacy means surviving the continued subjection of one's humanity within the narrow constraints of public comportment that will produce the 'good feelings' of pathos and social order in hegemonic society, and that life as a cultural producer under those same conditions means balancing one's responsibilities as a participant in the aforementioned systems with the ceaseless question of *how am I gonna pay my rent?*

The following conversation between Vivek Shraya and I took place in the summer of 2020, in the midst of a global pandemic, during an international uprising under the banner of Black Lives Matter. This moment of upheaval and lockdown left the material underpinnings of state violence exposed to an unusual extent, laying a groundwork for our discussion on the form and function of public representations of racialized trauma, grief, resilience, and joy.

(Note: interview has been edited for clarity and length.)

* * *

Vivek Shraya: I think for me, one of the things that I'm really drawn to are quote unquote "difficult emotions." And part of that is because, as I have grown into an adult and had to encounter the reality that with most difficult—and again I'm saying difficult in quotation marks—or negative emotions, that the only way to really get through them or work through them or survive them is to actually acknowledge them. That for me personally, pushing something down or denying a particular feeling has actually made my circumstances more difficult. And so whether it's tackling fear or anger or jealousy—again, emotions that generally are seen as negative, or emotions that I would say that are, [or] can be seen as contrary to the expectations of resilience that are projected upon or expected of marginalized people and marginalized artists—they, to me, feel necessary to confront, necessary to reclaim, even if only to be able to move forward. And by move forward I mean, you know, live.

Pansee Atta: Absolutely. And it's interesting because there's this public-facing aspect of your practice, but the work you do is central to your own actual personal survival and your own resilience as well.

Shraya: Definitely, definitely. I mean, I pull so much from my own life experience in my art. And again, I think that one of the ways in which I've tried to support the communities that I'm part of has been to try to address or own some of these difficult emotions. So, for example, my band [with] my brother, *Too Attached*, we wrote and recorded our last album, *Angry*, around the time that Trump was elected, and obviously the conversations around anger and people of color are not new ones. You know, the expectation that we keep our anger to ourselves, the expectation for Black people, Black women, to be polite, I think that these are all things that we thought about when we wrote our album and decided that we wanted to create an album that people of color could put on in their bedrooms and be mad and for that to be a welcomed emotion as opposed to having to store it and put it somewhere else or find the right space to express anger. And even with our live shows, we always introduce the songs by saying: "This is a space for you to be mad. We welcome your rage here."

Atta: Mm hmm. There's this real community building aspect to expressing [the fact] that it's not always about resilience or hope or these positive feelings. Sometimes, centering work around the more negative or the more difficult emotions ends up being a kind of community building process too.

Shraya: Totally. Like even I wrote a book a few years ago called *I'm Afraid of Men*. And I remember having so many conversations with marginalized people just saying how thrilled they were to have a space where they could say that they were afraid. And one of the things I really tried to push forward with that project is, again, this way that marginalized people are expected to be courageous, right? Like, one of the things I hear as a trans artist is like, "You're so brave, you're so courageous," and to admit fear is in some ways to say "I'm not always brave, I'm not always courageous. I'm actually scared shitless." But I would like to position the naming of fear as a form of resilience in and of itself, that resilience doesn't have to just look like, "Ah, I'm gonna pick myself up and move through the world with a smile." Resilience can also look like "I don't know how to get through this world, I might just stay in bed today because I'm terrified." And to me, that feels just as important as a form of resilience.

Atta: Absolutely, yeah. And it sounds like part of it is also about pushing back against expectations around how to feel, like there's some feelings that are rendered as being more acceptable than others. And saying "I'm actually going to feel differently about this" when you have a public facing persona, that can be problematic [or] challenging.

Shraya: I mean, during the pandemic I've had to tell any organizer who's invited me to do an event, "I just want to be really transparent that if I get us to this sort of quintessential, you know, 'how are you managing the pandemic?', that I will be answering in a very honest way that involves talking about being depressed and my mental health, and I am unable to answer in a way that involves, you know, 'this has been an opportunity to reflect and to make bread'" and again, I know I'm saying that in a sort-of teasing way, but if anything, I'm envious of the quote unquote "resilience" I see around me, but it feels important to be, once again, honest about where I'm at, if only to try to create space for others who I know are also seeing the same forms of quote unquote "resilience" in their social media and feeling like "what's wrong with me, why don't I have the capacity to be a human anymore?" So, yes, I think to answer your question, I think it really is about giving space to unpopular emotions.

Atta: So much of it is this push to just express that your capacity has still not diminished despite everything being on fire everywhere in the world. It seems like that's bound up with the same questions around labor, and the expectation to perform a certain kind of positivity that's linked with our willingness and our ability to keep *doing*, to keep outputting work, to keep being productive…

Shraya: Which is bananas when you think about it, right? That's just… yeah, it's bananas and yet I've been putting that pressure on myself as well. I'm like, "What's wrong with me? Why don't I feel like myself? Why am I not feeling creative?"

Atta: Yeah. Which is interesting because I think that links as well to the ambivalence you've also expressed about centering work around those same negative feelings because of the idea that arts institutions will sometimes only make space for narratives around BIPOC misery, and sometimes that can be the only space that's around, and so on both sides, it seems like it's driven by these kinds of economic- or labor-based expectations…

Shraya: Totally! Like last year, I put out *Trauma Clown* and *Death Threat*, a comic book about being harassed online. They sort of landed at the same time and I think it was a little confusing to some people because they're like, "Wait a second. In one project, you're critiquing the pressures that BIPOC artists are under by audiences and institutions to create work that centers trauma and only trauma, and then simultaneously you're putting out a comic book about hate mail. Make up your mind, which one is it?" And I mean, I guess the thing is, for me, so much of it has to do with choice. I think that POC artists should have the freedom to express whatever we choose in our work, and if it is, to use your language, our misery, or if it is our trauma, or if it is our rage, you know, I want us to have that space. But I also feel like we deserve the space to write about the family dynamics in a suburb in an unnamed city in America. Like, that's not *my* dream, but I'm just saying I feel like it's so important that BIPOC artists just have a range of options and that we're able to choose.

And unfortunately, diversity in the arts often looks like "let's have a BIPOC person educate us on this panel," or "let's only support, publish, disseminate work by POC artists that are talking about how difficult their lives are." And so what that does is there's this huge onus on disclosure. And I again, to use my own example, when I was writing *I'm Afraid of Men* it was around the #MeToo moment and I felt like, "Am I allowed to write this book if I don't disclose an experience of sexual violence? Don't I have a responsibility with a title like *I'm Afraid of Men* to disclose, you know, something catastrophic?" There becomes this sort of pressure to perform pain, and I see this on social media a lot. And again, this isn't a critique of artists who choose to do this. But sometimes I wonder how much of it is coming from a place of "If I don't disclose how much pain I'm in, I'm not going to have support for my art," and I think that's really troublesome. And on the flip side of that equation, I sometimes feel, as someone who's a little bit more cautious about what I share online versus my art, sometimes I feel like if I'm not performing pain on the internet, that my work is also not taken seriously, that my *humanity* is also not taken seriously. You know, there's an assumption about me as a human, that I just run around and get blowouts and take selfies all day. And believe me, *I wish*, but that is *so* not the case. So much of that assumption comes from the fact that while there's certainly pain and trauma in my work, my online presence, I have a very different approach. And so, there's so many ways in which the pressure for BIPOC artists to share our pain, and the choice *to* and the choice *not to* have impacts on not only our careers, but our humanity.

Atta: Yeah, that's so much of it. There's also this top-down pressure from either funding bodies or arts institutions or audiences to consume what's most comfortable and what's least challenging. And sometimes that's just a performance of positivity and resilience and strength, and sometimes that's just the entrenchment of more

BIPOC trauma because that's what's most rewarded by those same institutions.

Shraya: Absolutely. And, I mean, I don't begrudge anyone for saying yes to those kinds of opportunities, because, you know, we need to make money, right? So yeah, I think it becomes a very, very complicated equation. And when you have gobs of debt, and you have rent and whatever your economic circumstances, it becomes very challenging to make quote unquote "authentic choices"—whatever that means—in your career.

[...]

Atta: Yeah, the way that this has played out for me once: I was in a seminar where I was talking about my work and the way that it relates to my identity and the politics of being an Arab and a Muslim, a first generation immigrant in the post-9/11 world and all those things. But the professor in that course was like, "Well, what kind of work are you gonna make once the US stops bombing the Middle East?" I don't know, I'm just gonna have to keep my fingers crossed that the ongoing imperialism in my place of origin continues, I guess? There seems to be this implicit understanding that the consumption of this continuous re-traumatization is what's desired since once that stops then you're going to be out of a job...

Shraya: Yeah, there's this part of my novel where the character talks a bit about what she refers to as the diversity stock market, and refers to younger artists and as she worries, "How many of them are just sort of anxious about their stock plummeting?" And I think that that's something I definitely see, where it's like, what's the trendy social issue this month or this year that will cause an uptick in interest in in people's work?

[...]

Atta: Yeah. Like in *Death Threat*, you're, like you said, taking the piss out of these letters, then you're robbing it of its power to some extent. But you were saying "If I had to write a grant about it, I'd have to talk about how difficult and traumatic this was, and that's maybe granting it more power." So I wonder if the form with which the subjects are presented is also part of it.

Shraya: I think that's definitely part of it. And I mean, I had this conversation with so many of my BIPOC friends. Are you in Canada?

Atta: Yeah, I'm in Ottawa right now.

Shraya: Okay. Yeah, so I mean, I don't know if you've personally ever applied for an arts grant before, but there does feel like there's this sort of disclosure that's expected. And I've had more success with grant applications if I've disclosed a lot more in terms of hardship and barriers and oppression. And it feels like that's what the jury wants to hear sometimes. And that feels challenging because when I pitched *Death Threat* to my publisher, I did it over the phone, and I pitched in a very cheeky kind of way, as opposed to, like you said, if I was writing a grant application, I feel like I would have had to have been like, you know, "the harrowing experience that I've had, writing a comic book would be a means to reclaim my narrative as a transgender person of color...', like, it's just a different kind of approach. And again, in fairness, no jury member has ever sat me down, or no granting body has ever sat me down, and been like "you must trauma clown in these applications." And I know that there's a lot of factors into why certain things get grants and why they don't, but I will say that if I map out my quote unquote "success" in relation to granting bodies, there is a correlation there that feels hard to ignore.

Atta: Yeah, I mean, you were talking about the audience earlier, and the inevitability of thinking of what audiences will react in certain ways to. But also, grant applications are a specific genre of writing with their own very specific audience, and that audience is most often established arts industry professionals, and so you always end up having to write with that audience in mind. And so it ends up being like, "what will that audience be most able to consume and appreciate?"

Shraya: Yeah, exactly [...] Yeah. I don't know. It's been really interesting, I put out a novel in April called *The Subtweet*. And I really see some of the projects I put up this year as my effort to sort of move a bit away from the ways in which trauma or oppression has been so deeply centered in my work. And in fairness, certainly gender and sexism and racism are at the core of *The Subtweet* as well, but you know, the book is called *The Subtweet*, for instance, as opposed to, let's say, *Death Threat* or *I'm Afraid of Men*. And one of the things that I've really noticed with the book is, I would say, almost for the first time in my career, the bulk of the questions I'm getting asked are about the craft and the mechanism and the character development and the layout and the narrative arc. And I was saying to my partner, I feel this is the first project, I don't know, maybe *ever* in my career where I feel like I'm being treated like an artist, as opposed to an educator, as opposed to a teacher of some kind. And I say that as someone who *is* an educator, but I do think that art can be a powerful tool to teach, but the unfortunate part of exposing trauma in my work—whether by choice or not—has been that when I put out an album called *Part-time Woman* that features an orchestra and a choir and backup vocalist, I get questions like "So what would you tell a parent who has a trans child?" And again, happy to answer the question. But curious if anyone actually listened to the album? Or you know, I put out a book called *even this page is white* that uses a range of different kinds of poetry styles and yet the number one question I get asked is "So how do you recommend being an ally? What would you recommend to white people in terms of allyship?" and I'm like, "Read the book." And so, to me, it's just been really eye opening and freeing to put out a project that still engages with social issues, but because of, to your point, perhaps the packaging of a novel and also because the politic is arguably less at the forefront, it means that I get to be seen as an artist. And to me, as an artist, there's something quite essential and lovely about that experience. I'm a multidisciplinary artist, I jump all over the place, but I basically have been, like, "maybe just, like, build a home in novels," and maybe it's the only place that I'm going to get taken seriously as an artist as opposed to an educator.

* * *

In this discussion, Shraya contests the oft-reiterated supposition of positive affect's normativity. Lisa Duggan and José Muñoz respectively state that "[a]s a queer feminist anti-imperialist and utterly contrary and cranky leftist, I have my doubts about the political valences of hope. I'm suspicious of it. I associate it with normative prescriptions about the future I *ought* to want[,]" reminding us that "[w]e cannot discount the importance of the paranoid schizoid positions and its pleasures—its negative force as an anti-normative resource for queer existence" (Duggan and Muñoz 2009, pp. 276–281, see also Muñoz 2006a, p. 675). Sara Ahmed posits the 'happy object' as one that exists in proximity to social norms that are moralized as both the source and trajectory of happiness, the rejection of which renders one into an 'unhappy object' whose own supposed unhappiness is understood in turn as the source of unhappiness in others (Ahmed 1984, 2010). Earlier still, in the context of racialized and gendered labor, Arlie Hochschild's framework of "feeling rules" draws attention to the proscription of Black anger in the workplace, but glosses over the hyper-visibility of racialized trauma and misery in mass media, despite the production of those images as a site of emotional labor in its own right (Hochschild 1983, pp. 113–114).

Shraya's practice acknowledges and embraces the exigencies of anger and trauma in communities of marginalized peoples; she reiterates that:

> Whether it's tackling fear or anger or jealousy—again, emotions that generally are seen as negative, or emotions that I would say that are, [or] can be seen as contrary to the expectations of resilience that are projected upon or expected of marginalized people and marginalized artists—they, to me, feel necessary to confront, necessary to reclaim, even if only to be able to move forward. And by move forward I mean, you know, live.

But while normative performances of happiness, gratitude, and resilience are certainly weaponized as part of capitalist, White supremacist, and cis-heteropatriarchal social structures, the cultural sector demands and consumes racial trauma as part of its own multi-billion dollar moral economy. Kara Brown notes the normativity and commercialization of Black performances of negative affect: "When movies about slavery or, more broadly, other types of violence against Black people are the only types of films regularly deemed 'important' and 'good' by white people, you wonder if white audiences are only capable of lauding a story where Black people are subservient" (Brown 2016). Images of racialized misery and oppression abound; in fact, they arguably predominate in arts and mass media. Shraya draws attention to the imbrication of the social, economic, and psychic dimensions of the unending public performance of negative affect on artists of color:

> There becomes this sort of pressure to perform pain [...] sometimes I wonder how much of it is coming from a place of "If I don't disclose how much pain I'm in, I'm not going to have support for my art," and I think that's really troublesome. And on the flip side of that equation, I sometimes feel, as someone who's a little bit more cautious about what I share online versus my art, sometimes I feel like if I'm not performing pain on the internet, that my work is also not taken seriously, that my *humanity* is also not taken seriously.

That bad feelings can be made productive is not a new observation; Deborah Gould remarks: "From very early on in ACT UP when AIDS activists wondered, 'How do we turn grief into anger? How do we turn people's rage into action?'" (Gould et al. 2019, p.100). Similarly, Lauren Berlant's work with "Feel Tank" strives to reframe negative political emotions (such as "detachment, numbness, vagueness, confusion, bravado, exhaustion, apathy, discontent, coolness, hopelessness, and ambivalence") as a mode of criticality, a valence of social and political attachment to be interrogated rather than denied (Berlant 2004, pp. 450–451, see also Cvetkovich 2012, pp. 1–3, Ngai 2005, pp. 2–4).

The argument arising from Shraya's observation here is not that a critical socio-economy of queer, Brown negative affect should shun these dimensions of affective sociality and action; rather that *our subjectivities are teleologically constrained even within the critical formulations that accommodate negative affect.* This is to say that the cases for positive and negative affective modes of sociality are made by their respective capacities to *produce*: 'good' feelings in White audiences, comfort in our colleagues, positive social change in the communities to which we belong, etc. The effect of this is the continued privatization of our inner lives, an affective neoliberalism that cannibalizes expressions of the same trauma it inflicts.

Shraya's call to open up the sphere of artistic possibility for queer BIPOC artists should in this context be understood not as a call to evade political responsibility and retreat into the comfort of a compulsory performance of positive affect; rather, it is a defense of a radical politics of refusal, one that withholds the normative image of the 'trauma clown', substituting in its stead creative output that insists on the fullness of BIPOC humanity and the nuance of queer and trans life.

It is in this context that Shraya's rejection of the imperative to 'educate' can be understood; *of course* her practice remains pedagogically engaged with the realities of ongoing oppression. Rather, it is a rejection of inequitable and traumatic working conditions, of the demand to continuously diminish the breadth of one's humanity into soundbites that produce 'good feelings', to repeatedly relive violence as part of a moralized imperative to *serve*.

Shraya's desire for the novel form is a desire to explore the entirety of affect's terrain, her own and that of her characters. It is a desire to no longer be called on to unceasingly utilize her trauma as a means of aiding privileged audiences in recognizing her humanity. It is a desire to be unburdened from affect's *telos* in the form of compulsory community service. The public performance of personal and communal trauma is hard work, and, like all of us, Shraya has been *feeling unproductive*.

* * *

Vivek Shraya: Just to circle [back] quickly to the notion of teaching and not wanting to teach: the truth is, I think one of the reasons why I struggle so much is because I do feel a social responsibility to use my platform to bring awareness, to educate... and so, I think some artists are really good about drawing that line of like, "educate yourself, I'm not here to educate you" and I find that very difficult. I totally respect that perspective in that position, but simultaneously, as a non-Black or non-Indigenous person of color, or someone who has a certain kind of class privilege, I do feel a responsibility to use those privileges, to teach where possible. And so I think that, again, I'm definitely part of this equation because I don't always have clear boundaries in terms of like, "this is my art, I won't educate you." If you were to see me at a panel or whatever, for the most part, I try to be quite forthcoming, and when I

> do get questions around allyship and whatnot, I definitely feel compelled to answer. And yeah, I think it's hard. It's hard for me to know. I struggle with drawing that line.

References

Ahmed, Sara. 1984. Happy Objects. In *The Affect Theory Reader*, ed. Melissa Gregg and Gregory J. Seigworth, 30–50. Durham: Duke University Press.

Ahmed, Sara. 2010. *The Promise of Happiness*. Durham: Duke University Press.

Berlant, Lauren. 2004. Critical Inquiry, Affirmative Culture. *Critical Inquiry* 30 (2): 445–451.

Brown, Kara. 2016. I'm So Damn Tired of Slave Movies. *Jezebel*, 27 January. https://jezebel.com/im-so-damn-tired-of-slave-movies-1755250873.

Cvetkovich, Ann. 2012. *Depression: A Public Feeling*. Durham: Duke University Press.

Duggan, Lisa, and José Esteban. Muñoz. 2009. Hope and Hopelessness: A Dialogue. *Women and Performance* 19 (2): 275–283.

Gould, Deborah, Rory Barron, Brittany Frodge, and Robby Hardesty. 2019. Affect and Activism: An Interview with Deborah Gould. *DisClosure: A Journal of Social Theory* 28 (1): 95–108.

Hochschild, Arlie Russell. 1983. *The Managed Heart: The Commercialization Human of Feeling*. Berkley and Los Angeles: University of California Press.

Muñoz, José Esteban. 2006a. Feeling Brown, Feeling down: Latina Affect, the Performativity of Race, and the Depressive Position. *Signs: Journal of Women in Culture and Society* 31 (3): 675–688.

———. 2006b. The Vulnerability Artist: Nao Bustamante And the Sad Beauty of Reparation. *Women and Performance* 16 (2): 191–200.

Ngai, Sianne. 2005. *Ugly Feelings*. Cambridge: Harvard University Press.

CHAPTER 11

I Want to Be a Seashell, I Want to Be a Mold, I Want to Be a Spirit

Francesca Ekwuyasi

This essay is named after Noboru Kawazoe's essay of the same title in the Metabolist Manifesto Metabolism: The Proposals for New Urbanism. *Metabolism was a post-World War II Japanese architectural movement that combined ideas about architecture with organic biological growth during the reconstruction of large cities. I came across the quote, "I want to be a seashell, I want to be a mold, I want to be a spirit," at a group art show called "Gut Feelings" (Dalhousie Art Gallery, Kjipuktuk/Halifax, Nova Scotia) in which interdisciplinary artist, Lou Sheppard, rendered the quote in black ink on brown paper. The words deeply resonate with the longing—at the height of my depression—to cease to exist as myself; to live as something else beautiful, useful, and perhaps mute.*

"Are you a slut for words?" my friend, Frank, asks me via text, "like do you love words?"

"I'm a slut for words," I reply.

The correction of this chapter can be found under https://doi.org/10.1007/978-3-030-80554-8_16

F. Ekwuyasi (✉)
Lagos, Nigeria

J. Hollenbach and R. A. McDonald (eds.), *Re/Imagining Depression*, https://doi.org/10.1007/978-3-030-80554-8_11

On the phone the next day, Frank tells me they came upon the word ***quixotic*** and thought of me.

Quix·ot·ic
/kwikˈsädik/
adjective
Exceedingly idealistic, unrealistic, and impractical.

The word is derived from Miguel de Cervantes' *The Ingenious Gentleman Don Quixote of La Mancha* (1605; 1615). The protagonist, Alonso Quixano, a nobleman from La Mancha who loses his mind after reading many chivalric romances, decides to become a knight-errant and restore chivalry in service to his nation. Don Quixote, hit with a potent brew of optimism or delusion—or both, fails to see the world as it is; instead, he lives out his imagined story of knighthood and nobility.

Frank thinks I'm irrationally optimistic, overly idealistic about the world, about people, about love, perhaps even verging on delusional. I cannot argue that they are entirely wrong; I believe that the stories we tell ourselves and each other shape our realities, and I don't mean this in a witchy, supernatural way. No, I mean it more in the sci-fi Matrix way, wherein material worlds are made and re-made through ideas. Regardless, on my best days, I choose a doggedly optimistic quixotic path; I tell myself stories about the world full of loving possibilities, stories about the inevitability of sunrise, of the sheer blissful magic of bees, and maggots, and slugs, and spiders.

The thing is that my brain seems to like extremes: so as intense or Pollyannaish as my optimism can come across, there is an equal and opposite version that sometimes seizes me. When I wake up crying for the fourth day in a row with an unfocused dread gnawing away at my chest, I know that I have been seized. This descent was not swift (it never is); for me, there are always material conditions that stitch the claws that grasp me. In retrospect, I often imagine it as a setup: nothing sinister, more like Jenga, or the proverbial last straw on camel's broken back. What I mean is that when I was diagnosed with depression a few years ago, the psychologist explained that it made sense that I was depressed. *I had just moved countries, and the seasonal shift was likely doing a number on me; I was away from family, adjusting to grad school, must be so lonely, must feel totally out of control.* At the time, I sought to control the things I could; I dove into my coursework and starved myself.

As a child, I lost my father, grandfather, and eldest brother in six consecutive years—material conditions for the immense sadness that coloured my childhood. Idiosyncratic yet not uncommon family dynamics rendered me a lonely teenager and gifted me with many opportunities to explore solitude. Stories, books, and imagination became my most consistent companions; now, I appreciate how they shaped me.

Now I also appreciate that my identities and the particular ways they intersect in this precise configuration of the global sociopolitical climate are material conditions for my present state of depression. I exist and I am Black; I cannot honestly write about my experiences of depression without bringing up racism, without bringing up misogynoir, a term created by Moya Bailey, a queer Black feminist scholar, "to express the specific ways in which Black women (cis and trans) are targeted within popular culture. The term is a combination of misogyny, the hatred of women and noir, which means black but also carries film and media connotations. It is the particular amalgamation of anti-black racism and misogyny in popular media and culture that targets black trans and cis women" (2013, p. 26). I apply this term to contextualize my personal experiences of racism + misogyny.

The trouble is that I don't want to talk about misogynoir, I don't want to talk about the historic, systemic, and institutional machinations that allow and profit off the dehumanisation of Black women. I don't want to think in theories—to recognize the constellational roots such as the Transatlantic slave trade, colonisation, "cisnormative heteronormative imperialist white supremacist capitalist patriarchy" (Laverne Cox, 14 November 2015)—and symptoms of global anti-Blackness. But I cannot unknow what I know (there's no going back to sleep once you take the red pill). So here's some more things I know: one hundred and sixty-nine years after Sojourner Truth extemporaneously delivered the speech *Ain't I a Woman,* particularly this line "*Dat man ober dar say dat women needs to be helped into carriages, and lifted over ditches, and to have de best place eberywhar. Nobody eber helps me into carriages or ober mud-puddles, or gives me any best place. -And ar'n't I a woman?*" from Frances Gage's inaccurate version of the Truth's speech printed in the April 1863 Issue of the *New York Independent*, I write affirmations to myself, I tell myself that I am worthy and deserving of gentleness, of sweetness, of being protected, and comforted. I think of a horrific thing (I won't name the specific horrific thing that crosses my mind because there's no need to spread the horror, but I will mention that, anecdotally—from my personal experiences of and interactions with social media—there seems to be a normalisation of sharing graphic scenes of revolting violence against Black people, Black women and girls). And it hurts. It makes me ever more certain that I must grind these affirmations into my mind, integrate them, because if I were to concede to what dominant culture insists upon, then I would be convinced that sweetness, tenderness, and acts of chivalry are reserved neither for me nor folks who look like me.

I am also queer, an immigrant—the only person in my biological family living in Canada, a woman; all of which comes with considerable amounts of marginality in a world rife with injustice. I am living in a global pandemic. My home country, Nigeria, is currently undergoing something akin to a revolution, hopefully. Thousands of people gathered in protest against the country's corruption and police brutality in October, the month of Nigeria's sixtieth independence anniversary. These protests, primarily led by young people, called for abolishing Nigeria's Special Anti-Robbery Squad, known as SARS, which has been known to make unlawful arrests and harassment, extortion, rape, torture, and murder. On 20 October 2020, the Nigerian military opened fire at the Lekki tollgate plaza in Lagos, killing thirty-eight protesters, in what was soon called "the Lekki Massacre." The government has attempted to curtail these protests by instating a curfew and suppressing the media by releasing guidelines that effectively penalize news outlets that cover the demonstrations. The world is grieving, kicking, screaming, writhing into a potential revolution.

But really is anyone undisturbed at the state of the world at the moment? Is anyone's mental health—regardless of identity—flourishing? No, really, show me a single person who is unaffected (who isn't completely blinded by their privilege.)

I know there is no need to justify how a person might come upon depression. Material conditions aside, there's also just the brain and its particular chemistry to account for. However, I mention these aspects of my identities and how they inform my experience of depression to illustrate how they also speak to my craft, which relates to the primary way I move through it—the same way I move through everything: by writing. I write about being alive, being an animal, being human—which, for me, means being a Black woman, a queer person, an immigrant. I write about experiencing the full depth and breadth of emotion, which, for me, has included despair, grief, sorrow, apathy alongside immeasurable joy, pleasure, and fulfillment.

Writing these words has taken me three times longer than it would have during a more balanced season. And yet, because I'm a slut for words, because I'm quixotic, I tell myself a story in which I am the courageous protagonist. Even though I have a penchant for escapism, and sometimes long to disappear, to be elsewhere, or to cease to exist altogether, to feel nothing—simultaneously my worst fear and, yet sometimes, the very thing I desire most. Even though my depression is a melodramatic teen, excessive, demanding, I must ride it out, must give her the attention she craves. Even in the throes of it, I know that my art will save me. I am romantic; I know that my craft will make this pain bearable, perhaps even fruitful. This is why I always return to writing, to making. I am on a hero's journey; I will make meaning of all this shit! It will be worthwhile in the end.

References

Bailey, Moya Zakia. 2013. *Race, Region, and Gender in Early Emory School of Medicine Yearbooks*. Doctoral dissertation, Emory University, Atlanta, GA, USA.

Cox, Laverne. 2015. Actually Its Cisnormative Heteronormative Imperialist White Supremist Capitalist Patriarchy My Spin on @bellhooks. @Lavernecox. Twitter, 14 November. https://twitter.com/Lavernecox/status/665595357288640513.

N.D. Compare the Speeches. *The Sojourner Truth Project*. Retrieved 20 November 2020. https://www.thesojournertruthproject.com/compare-the-speeches.

CHAPTER 12

Being Sita: Gayathri Ramprasad's *Shadows in the Sun*

Sabrina Reed

Gayathri Ramprasad's memoir, *Shadows in the Sun: Healing from Depression and Finding the Light Within* (2014b), recounts her experiences with severe depression, from its onset through to how she learned to mitigate her symptoms and embrace a life which, though not entirely free of mental illness, was more fulfilling than she had previously thought possible. Ramprasad attributes her depression to numerous factors, both cultural and hereditary, but she believes her symptoms were exacerbated by what she calls "the diametric cultural forces that tug and tear at [her] very core" (2014b, p. 179). Growing up in Bangalore, India, Ramprasad was torn between her father's love for all things American and her mother's Hindu beliefs and desire to mold her daughter into a paragon of traditional womanhood. This tension came to the fore during her adolescence in 1970s India. Ramprasad writes, "While my mother's goal is to groom me into a god-fearing domestic diva, my father's vision is for me

S. Reed (✉)
Department of English, Languages, and Cultures, Mount Royal University, Calgary, AB, Canada
e-mail: sreed@mtroyal.ca

J. Hollenbach and R. A. McDonald (eds.), *Re/Imagining Depression*,
https://doi.org/10.1007/978-3-030-80554-8_12

to become a modern, ambitious woman who is unafraid to follow her dreams. My life, therefore, becomes a mixture of mantras and miniskirts—a dizzying blend of two cultures, two continents, worlds apart" (2014b, p. 24).

After an adolescence in which she tried to balance her need for independence with the societal constraints often placed on South Asian women, a traumatic incident at age eighteen triggered what she calls her "tryst with terror" (2014b, p. 177), the onset of severe anxiety and depression. At twenty-two, after an arranged marriage to a South Asian man already residing in the United States, Ramprasad moved to the country of her father's dreams, yet her depression and alienation, her feeling of being caught between two cultures, continued. As one of her therapists says to her, "the interpersonal skills you needed to survive in India are almost opposite of the skills you need to thrive in America" (2014b, p. 179). Desiring independence yet tied to South Asian ideals of womanhood, missing her family while savoring her solitary life in America, Ramprasad experiences alienation in both her home and adopted countries, and this alienation is a major contributor to her mental illness. In her search to alleviate her symptoms, Ramprasad embraces aspects of American/European psychotherapy, but she also returns to her roots, learning to value Indian yogic practices.

In this chapter I will read Ramprasad's memoir of depression through the lens of Carl Elliott's analysis of alienation in American society. In his essay, "Pursued by Happiness and Beaten Senseless: Prozac and the American Dream," Carl Elliott writes, "Alienation generally describes an incongruity between the self and external structures of meaning—a lack of fit between the way you are and the way you are expected to be" (2004, p. 129). Though Elliott cautions against conflating alienation with depression, since the two conditions "do not necessarily go hand in hand," he recognizes that "alienation of any type might go together with depression" because estrangement from the norms that are supposed to make one happy can leave one feeling depressed (2004, p. 133). Elliott objects to over-prescription of SSRIs such as Prozac because, when depression stems from alienation, curing the symptoms of depression without examining their root cause might be like placing a bandage on a cancer that needs to be excised. In the sense that depression might encourage individuals to examine the roots of their unhappiness in an effort to alleviate psychic pain, depression can be a positive step on the road to identifying the circumstances which caused an individual to feel alienated in the first place. Although Ramprasad does not discount the agony of severe depression, her narrative reflects Elliott's theories in that it shows how depression can grow from alienation, and how it can, in that sense, be a valuable awakening to unsatisfactory life conditions that require change.

As a bioethicist and medical doctor, Carl Elliott's work has focused on the intersections between American society's increasing infatuation with enhancement technologies—"medical technology [used] not merely to cure or control illness but to enhance a person's appearance, personality, or capacities (e.g., stimulants to improve concentration, growth hormone to increase height, antidepressants for shyness, and so on)"—and medical ethics (2011, p. 364). Asking why American culture has so wholeheartedly embraced such technologies, Elliott posits that the answer lies in three areas: "the importance of social recognition, the ethics of authenticity, and the rise of instrumental reason" (2011, p. 366).

According to Elliott, "for many Westerners today, it is very important that others recognize and respect them for who they are as individuals" rather than for the generic categories—education, job type, class—they represent (2011, p. 366). Stigmatized qualities such as racialized features, shyness, and old age all lessen the chance that one's individual being will be judged acceptable, that one will achieve desired social recognition, and thus "much of the moral justification for prescribing enhancement drugs comes from the desire to remedy this kind of shame" (2011, p. 367). The same logic applies to physical interventions such as cosmetic surgery. Even though enhancements such as taking anxiolytics to reduce shyness or rhinoplasty to produce a Greco-Roman profile can be said to change an individual's mental or physical identity, making that person less "authentic," Elliott notes, following Peter Kramer's comments in *Listening to Prozac,* that enhancements are often perceived as making patients more like themselves, "or putting them in touch with themselves, or showing them a part of themselves that was previously hidden from them" (2011, p. 369).

Furthermore, Western society's preference for individualized selves over communal identities manifests as an ethics of authenticity, or a belief in the imperative of finding one's true self, unadulterated by convention or social expectations. Referring to the ideas of philosopher Charles Taylor, Elliott writes of how a commitment to authenticity implies "there is something morally important about being true to yourself as an individual and that a meaningful life involves getting in touch with your own inner depths" (2011, p. 369). Theoretically, enhancement technologies can help a person reveal their "true" identity. For example, anxious people may feel that anxiolytic drugs allow them to access their hidden, more outgoing (and in American Society, more valued) personality traits (2011, pp. 368–370). Finally, Western society embraces enhancement technologies because of what Charles Taylor calls "instrumental reason": "By instrumental reason I mean the kind of rationality we draw on when we calculate the most economical application of means to a given end" (as quoted in Elliott 2011, p. 371). Elliott elaborates, "Instrumental reason encourages us to see the world as a project to be shaped and used. … The value of the world is measured in terms of what it can give us" (2011, p. 371).

As readers of this chapter may have noticed, there are contradictions inherent in the above explanation of Americans' embrace of enhancement technologies: instrumental reason encourages a consumerist culture in which we engineer our happiness using the technologies available to us, but doing so makes our happiness our sole responsibility, even when we know, on some level, that social, spiritual, and environmental factors are largely outside our control. Lennard Davis, for example, critiques attitudes to depression, from the 1950s to the present, which assume that "when you are depressed, it is you who suffer and no one else. Depression isn't defined as a communal activity or one that results from a set of environmental circumstances that have become normalized to appear almost undetectable. Depression is never seen as a consequence of the multilayered exigencies of life in the postwar United States" (2013, p. 47). Similarly, in an insightful analysis of "Racism and Depression," Ann Cvetkovich asks "what kinds of therapy and social change could 'cure' the psychic fallout of colonialism and slavery across a range of generations and different kinds of people" (2012, p. 118).

Elliott writes, "the problems that enhancement technologies are intended to fix have social roots, and often these social roots are objectionable. Yet it feels easier to use technology to change the individual than to fix the social problems. Many people have soul-deadening jobs" and therefore "it is not hard to see why they are interested in stimulants. But the larger problem is their boring soul-deadening jobs" (2011, p. 373). Similarly, Elliott notes that individuals with racialized facial features may desire cosmetic surgery, but such surgery will not address the larger societal imperative to fight and eradicate racism (2011, p. 373). In fact, "the widespread use of the technologies simply reinforces the social norms whose damaging effects they are intended to remedy" (Elliott 2011, p. 367).

Elliott uses the suburbs as an example of the conundrum faced by American society. Wishing to establish a valuable identity by proving upward mobility and financial success, people moved to the suburbs in the 1950s and 60s, only to find that the experience was empty and that, in spite of having obtained material desires, they were still alienated and depressed. Following Susan Sontag and Robert Bellah, Elliott suggests that desire for social recognition encourages people to match or surpass the material status of their neighbors, but the search for status can lead to feelings of inauthenticity, since one is conforming to others' expectations rather than finding one's own unique and creative way of living (2003, pp. 132–140). In such circumstances, alienation, "a mismatch between the way you are living a life and the structures of meaning that tell you how to live a life" (Elliott 2004, p. 129), may set in.

To Elliott, and most relevant to Gayathri Ramprasad's *Shadows in the Sun*, sometimes alienation is both merited and necessary. A sense of alienation may, after all, cause one to ask why such a feeling exists, and to acknowledge that one is alienated for good reason. While enhancement technologies such as antidepressants can be used to reduce feelings of unhappiness and angst, Elliott and others, such as David Healy (1997, pp. 226–31) and Erik Parens (2004), worry that people may lose sight of the fact that "some external circumstances call for alienation" (Elliott 2004, p. 130). Elliott continues,

> Here is the key to the problem psychiatry has with a notion like alienation. The measure of psychiatric success is internal psychic well-being. The aim of psychiatry is (among other things) to get rid of anxieties, obsessions, compulsions, phobias, and various other barriers to good social functioning. Within this framework, where the measure of success is psychic well-being through good social functioning, alienation is something to be eliminated. It is a psychiatric complaint. It is a barrier to psychic well-being. Whereas what I want to suggest is that maybe psychic well-being is not everything. (p. 134)

Ramprasad says something similar in *Shadows in the Sun*, where she quotes Jiddu Krishnamurti and reminds her readers that "it is not a sign of good health to be well adjusted to a sick society" (2014b, p. 201). If, as Ramprasad suggests, her depression stems from unease with the constraints placed upon her as a South Asian woman, curing her depression without addressing its root causes might be counterproductive. Ramprasad eventually decides, "I no longer want to remain well adjusted to a sick society. I want to get well and live 'well adjusted' in a world that honors my truth and humanity" (p. 201).

In this regard, Ramprasad's analysis echoes recent studies which have examined the link between South Asian women's depression and structural oppression. Rao, Horton, and Raguram, for instance, write of how "the ancient Hindu Laws of Manu state that women are never independent; they are to be protected by their fathers when young, their husbands when married, and their sons in old age" (2012, p. 1968). In a culture where the advent of sex-selective abortion has changed the ratio of children under the age of six "from 976 girls per 1000 boys in 1961 to 914 girls per 1000 boys in 2011," it is unsurprising that there is a link between "the internalization of socially defined gender roles to the emergence of depressive symptoms in women, mediated by the constructs of shame and self-esteem" (Robitaille and Chatterjee 2016, p. 47; Rao et al. 2012, p. 1968). Although Ramprasad begins *Shadows in the Sun* with happy childhood memories of her family's celebration of Diwali, the Hindu festival marking "the triumph of good over evil, light over darkness," precursors of darker times appear even then. She is a dearly loved daughter, yet she knows that her brother has more privilege and a more important place in the family hierarchy (Ramprasad 2014b, p. 5).

Ramprasad also encounters an early example of how women are defined by their relationships to men. When Ramprasad's grandfather dies, her grandmother, "now a widow, is stripped of her *mangalsutra* (the wedding necklace), the *bindi* (the traditional red dot on her forehead), her toe rings, and the cluster of colorful bangles that had long adorned her hands—all sacred symbols of her married life" (2014b, p. 13). When her marital home is sold, she also loses her authority as head female in the household, a happening that Ramprasad says makes her own mother more content, since her mother is "no longer under the vigilance of her mother or mother-in-law" (2014b, p. 16).

Ramprasad grows up with mixed messages about her status as a woman. Unlike the fathers in most of the families in her neighborhood, Ramprasad's father, Appa, encourages his wife to eat at the family table rather than eating separately once others are finished, to do her own banking, and to have a say in family decision making. Appa loves all things American, and he thus believes that women can have more than a solely domestic existence. "Appa's temper tantrums," however, "are legendary in [the] family. So are his sullen retreats, but no one ever questions them" because they are seen "as a man's prerogative" (2014b, p. 43). (As an interesting aside, in her mid-twenties, Ramprasad learns of another explanation for her father's moodiness: he suffers from depression. However, because of the shame such a diagnosis would bring to the family, her father's moods were not discussed, even when Ramprasad began to exhibit symptoms of depression at age eighteen).

Meanwhile, Ramprasad's mother, Amma, works diligently to instill the skills and values which will make her daughters attractive and marriageable. "It was her fond hope," writes Ramprasad, "that her daughters would grow up to be like Sita, the revered epitome of Indian womanhood. She prayed that Chitra and I would evolve into pious, self-sacrificing, ever-loving women of grace" (2014b, p. 17). The Hindu epic, *The Ramayana,* tells of how Sita, the wife of the Hindu god Rama, is abducted by the evil demon Ravana. Although Rama rescues his consort, he fears that she may have succumbed to Ravana's sexual aggressions, and thus he repudiates her for potential impurity. Sita endures banishment and trial by fire in an attempt to prove her virtue, but when Rama still has doubts, Sita asks Mother Earth to swallow her into the ground. Raised to respect Sita's "virtues of stoic sacrifice," and to believe that "selflessness is a virtue and selfishness is a sin," Ramprasad experiences dissonance between the ideal of being Sita and her desire for autonomy (2014b, pp. 197, 173).

Unfortunately, society in 1970s India acts to quell Ramprasad's budding independence. When she cuts her hair, wears miniskirts, and plucks her eyebrows, her angry mother tells her that she "look[s] like a prostitute," and "the catcalls of strangers on the streets and the taunts of [her] classmates make [her] feel like a freak" (2014b, pp. 25, 26). In fact, Ramprasad continues, "Ever since I had emerged into puberty, I had become prey to boys and men alike," an observation borne out by an egregious action on the part of Gopal, a male classmate (p. 26). When Ramprasad declines to be his girlfriend, Gopal bribes college authorities to give her a failing grade in Mathematics, and Ramprasad, who now feels shame for disappointing *both* her parents, falls apart. Deeply angry, she dreams of confronting Gopal, but she understands her powerlessness in the face of masculine and economic privilege. She writes of her experience: "as a young woman born and raised in India, where men reign supreme, I realize I am helpless. I know any reaction from me, other than total submission, will only incite Gopal's rage further. I am fully aware that as a young man in India, with the means to bribe his way into anything he desires, Gopal has the power to not only deter me from graduating, but also to destroy my life" (2014b, p. 48). Events are made worse when Gopal brags that he plans to rape her on an upcoming school trip.

Although not diagnosed until much later, Ramprasad responds by becoming clinically depressed. She becomes exhausted, sleepless, and anxious, but her most distressing symptom is her inability to keep down food. Her symptoms are thus in keeping with research that shows depression in India, especially among women, often manifests through somatic indicators (Rao et al. 2012, p. 1967; Pereira et al. 2007, p. 209). In India, "Mental illness is still not well understood, often ignored, and considered a taboo" (Kishore et al. 2011, p. 325), and therefore individuals often present with somatic symptoms because "depressive symptoms affect the perceived social status of those who suffer from them in ways that somatic symptoms do not" (Raguram et al. 1996, p. 1048). Moreover, even when individuals request help, there are few resources to treat the illness. Almanzar et al. note, for instance, that India "only has approximately 5000 psychiatrists, which is equal to 1 psychiatrist per 200,000 people" (2014, p. 94). Ramprasad herself mentions that "there are a mere thirty-seven mental institutions to serve the country's population of 1.2 billion people—50 to 90 percent of people affected by mental illness, therefore, go untreated" (2014b, p. 156).

While Ramprasad and others examine the deficits in South Asian mental health systems, it is important to remember that any analysis needs to take into account India's colonial history. For example, Jain et al. note that before independence in 1947, deplorable "conditions in India's asylums became part of nationalist critiques of British rule" (2017, p. 43). In addition, although "the notion of a disturbed mind occurs in the oldest texts in South Asia, the *Vedas* and the *Upanishads*," traditional methods of dealing with mental illness have often been discredited and discounted by those who have been trained in European/American psychiatry (Jain et al. 2017, p. 41). After all, as Rao, Horton, and Raguram confirm, "consistent with Ayurvedic tradition, Indian ethno-medicine and philosophy do not subscribe to a Cartesian dualism that sees mind and body as distinct" (2012, p. 1967). Jain et al. write, "the history of psychiatry in India could thus be seen as a product of the colonial enterprise which constructed an alien illness narrative that was profoundly disconnected from the complex and diverse indigenous narratives in existence. This was accompanied by a delegitimization of the existing healing practices in the name of scientific and rational thought" (2017, pp. 54–55). In a strange way, Jain et al.'s analysis of the history of South Asian psychiatry mirrors Ramprasad's upbringing, with its conflicts between her mother's religious and social traditions and her father's love of American-style independence and progress.

Ramprasad's parents agree on one thing, however: their daughter's crying fits and chronic vomiting are self-indulgent. Several doctors, after all, have said that she is "a typical teenager—a drama queen asking for undue attention instead of navigating the road bumps of life with maturity and grace" (2014b, p. 45). But it is not surprising that Ramprasad's illness should manifest in a visceral rejection of food, as the book begins by describing the mouth-watering dishes eaten during the sacred festival of Diwali and continues by describing how Ramprasad's happiest moments with her mother, Amma, are in the kitchen. Food represents the best of Ramprasad's childhood, and she understands the importance of food at weddings, religious ceremonies, and in day-to-day life. As Amma reminds her, "It's not enough to know how to do calculus. It is also important to know how to cook" (2014b, p. 22). It makes sense, then, that when she is entrapped and angry after Gopal's harassment, Ramprasad rejects a key element of Indian society and a central aspect of her role as an Indian woman. Interestingly, as she describes further depressive episodes, Ramprasad returns to food: after her marriage, she cooks elaborate dinners for her husband and in-laws, and while experiencing post-partum depression after the birth of her first child, she still insists on having a birth celebration for which she cooks for three days straight, even though she cannot stomach what she has prepared.

Applying Carl Elliott's ideas to Ramprasad's mental illness, Ramprasad experiences alienation on two fronts. Having been encouraged by her father and her own instincts to assert her authenticity in terms of physical presentation and academic success, she collides with ideals for Indian womanhood which stress obedience and conformity. The once-headstrong daughter says nothing about Gopal's aggression because she fears her mother will "fault [her] for provoking Gopal's wrath by the way [she] dressed and behaved" (2014b, p. 48). In addition, Ramprasad feels alienated because she must act "normal" while she feels she is going mad. She writes, "Over the past year, my family and I have become experts at the *dance of denial,* pretending I am fine when I can barely function. And I have perfected the art of concealing my fears and tears behind a mask of makeup and smiles" (2014b, p. 51). Where before her illness, makeup was a form of self-expression and rebellion, it has now become a force for conformity.

Referencing the work of Marilyn Frye, Sara Ahmed writes, "to be oppressed requires that you show signs of happiness, signs of being or having been adjusted" (2010, p. 582). At this point in her life, Ramprasad has tried to gain recognition as an authentic individual, only to have her sense of self rejected by Gopal, her parents, and her doctors. Although on one level she knows she has reasons for being depressed (though she has not yet encountered the term), she does not want to bring shame on herself or her family. Ramprasad's mask of conformity "protects" her and lets her "function in the world," but it "sickens [her] to the very core of [her] mind, body, and soul" (2014b, 51). As Ahmed argues in "Killing Joy: Feminism and the History of Happiness," happiness can be a form of coercion, "a demand for agreement." When a woman—and Ahmed's examples are taken from European/American culture—disagrees with what her society believes should make her happy, she can be labelled a "killjoy," since her unhappiness may highlight injustices which others prefer to ignore. "We become alienated," writes Ahmed, "when we do not experience pleasure from proximity to objects that are attributed as being good" (2010, p. 580).

Such a situation occurs when, at age twenty-two, Ramprasad enters into an arranged marriage with Ram, a native of India now living and working in the United States. Her betrothal makes her "the luckiest girl in the world," for she has gained a prestigious marriage and a ticket to life in America (2014b, p. 62). Yet Ramprasad remains deeply troubled. Using the analogy of the *antarpata*, a muslin curtain which separates the couple during part of the marriage ceremony, Ramprasad writes, "I am terrified that, like the *antarpata*, my façade of normalcy will drop to unveil the crazy woman that I truly am" (2014b, p. 66). Again, her sense of self is split, for she knows that she is not the pristine wife Ram expects. Although writing about South Asian women with physical disabilities, Anita Ghai makes a point relevant to Ramprasad's experience: "the construction of daughter as a burden is rooted in the cultural milieu that looks at daughters as *Parai* (Other)" (2009, p. 300). Part of the duty of a girl's family is to raise her for marriage, with "the implicit understanding … that whatever you are giving will be perfect" (p. 300). This, in fact, is one reason why mental illness is particularly taboo for women in India: in a society in which depression is heavily stigmatized, mental illness can make women unmarriageable (Kishore et al., 2011, p. 328; Kulesza, Raguram and Rao, 2014, p. 74; Raguram et al., 1996, p. 1044). Since she feels far from perfect, Ramprasad is once again in a position where she must wear a mask and feel guilty for it. Add to this that she instinctively resents how she is "now expected to change magically into a dutiful daughter-in-law and serve [her] in-laws while waiting for [her] green card," and there are ample reasons for her illness to continue to plague her (2014b, p. 79).

Once she arrives in America, however, Ramprasad at first revels in the freedom she finds there and in her husband's insistence that "this is not India" and that he is "no God" (2014b, p. 101). She writes, "I cherish the newfound solitude of my life. I thrive on the freedom America affords me in forging a new life. The very things that made me a misfit in India help me acculturate in America—my independent spirit; my untraditional looks; my love for jeans, short hair, and makeup; my need for personal space; and above all, my fluency in English and lack of shyness" (2014b, p. 104). On one level, Ramprasad has pleased *both* her parents, since she has made an advantageous match, her mother's goal, and arrived in America, the dream of her father.

Yet Ramprasad has internalized her status as daughter and wife too well to be freed of her depression so easily. In fact, it is the next milestone of successful womanhood that leads to the return of her symptoms: the birth of her first child. Like many women, Ramprasad succumbs to postpartum depression, perhaps complicated in her case by resentment over the arrival of her in-laws. Although she would prefer her mother to visit her during her pregnancy, "the rules of patriarchy that bind [them] force [her] mother and [her] to honor the wishes of Ram and his parents" (2014b, p. 114). With her in-laws visiting, Ramprasad once again feels constrained by cultural expectations, and her health continues to decline.

Ramprasad is also plagued by others' assumptions that her illness is entirely her fault, not only on a personal but on a cosmic level. Many discourses on depression remove blame from the individual sufferer by adopting a causal model in which mental illness results from a combination of hereditary factors, chemical imbalance, and childhood trauma, rather than personal weakness or the perverse and selfish choices of the ill person. In *The Noonday Demon: An Atlas of Depression,* for example, Andrew Solomon writes of how "most depression mixes reactive and internal factors" and then, over the course of the book, goes on to discuss how depression can be attributed to, among other things, biochemical alterations in the brain, hereditary predisposition, traumatic incidents, poverty, and lack of light (2001, p. 62). Peter Kramer speaks of physiological and situational causes for depression in his book *Against Depression,* in which he also summarizes Kenneth Kendler's findings that major depressive episodes often follow stressful life events such as "being robbed or assaulted, facing housing or financial problems, losing a job or encountering serious work problems," and more (Kramer 2005, p. 138). Meanwhile, Gabor Maté's *In the Realm of Hungry Ghosts: Close Encounters with Addiction* states that "addicts are self-medicating conditions like depression, anxiety, post-traumatic stress or even ADHD" and that "a hurt is at the centre of *all* addictive behaviours" (2008, pp. 33, 36). In other words, for Solomon, Kramer, and Maté, all of whom have written popular accounts of mental illness, the factors which contribute to depression and addiction go far beyond the individuals themselves.

In contrast, the Hindu concept of *karma* suggests that sufferings (or benefits) in one's present life may be the result of merit or demerit accrued in previous lives. Someone, for example, who has abused his children in a past life may end up being re-born into an abusive household. A person who has lived a life of virtue, however, may be "born in a family of yogis rich in wisdom" (*The Bhagavad Gita* 6.42). In keeping with this concept, relatives tell Ramprasad to accept her suffering as retribution for sins in a past life (2014b, p. 210). Though Ramprasad tells her husband that she "will never accept this hell of a life as [her] karma," on another level the invocation of karma leaves her caught in "an inescapable web of guilt, hopelessness, and helplessness" (2014b, pp. 178, 210).

Although this essay cannot discuss every episode of depression described in *Shadows in the Sun*, it is significant that Ramprasad's worst depressive experiences begin when her mother writes to her saying: "Gayu, if only you prayed with a purer heart, you wouldn't be depressed the way you are." Following receipt of this letter, Ramprasad decides that her "only salvation is to follow in Goddess Sita's footsteps and retreat back in to the womb of [her] real mother—Mother Earth—just as Sita had done at the end of her trials in life" (2014b, p. 197). Ramprasad's husband comes home to discover his wife attempting to dig her own grave with her bare hands. After a stint in hospital, Ramprasad begins to recover, but soon after her return home, she has a miscarriage and again has to be hospitalized. Remembering her mother's words, "Gayu, a mother's state of mind is of utmost importance in the development of an unborn child," Ramprasad blames herself for the end of her pregnancy (2014b, p. 215).

Ramprasad's expression of suicidal thoughts prompts an incident that highlights the difficulties of imposing American/European psychiatric assumptions on those raised in other parts of the globe. Following hospital protocol, a nurse divests Ramprasad of all items that could be used for self-harm, including Ramprasad's *mangalsutra*, "the most sacred symbol of a Hindu marriage" which a woman only takes off upon widowhood or divorce (2014b, p. 217). While the nurse acts to protect her patient, she actually worsens Ramprasad's distress by symbolically dissolving her marriage. Already afraid that her husband will divorce her and take custody of their young daughter, Ramprasad feels completely bereft. She writes, "as an Indian woman, I had grown up believing there were only two measures of success: marriage and motherhood. Convinced that I have lost them both, I completely lose control" (2014b, p. 217).

Yet, having reached her lowest point, Ramprasad has a sudden insight that depression is not the result of bad karma or failure to pray. Moreover, she realizes she can no longer "be Sita," burying her true self under the mask of the ideal wife. To return to Carl Elliott's analogy of suburban life, Ramprasad has achieved what she says are the "only two measures of success" for a woman in India: "marriage and motherhood" (p. 217). And soon she also obtains the stereotypical symbol of American success: a giant house in the suburbs. Yet Elliott's observation proves true in that "once we see our homes not as an end in themselves, but as means to achieve self-fulfillment, then it is natural that any home will soon wear out, that we will always be looking for the next house, the one that has not been worn out yet" (Elliott 2003, pp. 150–51). The same can be said of marriage and motherhood in the sense that when the attributes which are supposed to make a woman happy are imposed by cultural norms, one might ask if they are really a guarantee of happiness or a capitulation to social expectations. If self-fulfillment is a cultural imperative, can it be as damaging as the imperative of conformity? Elliott writes, "Once self-fulfillment is hitched to the success of a human life, it comes perilously close to an obligation" (2003, p. 303). Ahmed says something similar: "When we feel pleasure from objects that are supposed to cause happiness, we are thus aligned. We are facing the right way. We become alienated when we do not experience pleasure from proximity to objects that are attributed as being good" (2010, p. 580).

This is not to say that Ramprasad dislikes motherhood or marriage in and of themselves; rather, she resents how these "goals" are supposed to make her feel completely fulfilled when she longs for more autonomy.

Ramprasad takes charge by actively challenging the behavioral dictates which have previously ruled her life: be silent, maintain the family honor, and do not reveal shameful secrets. Instead, she gets a job and later goes back to school, earning a second undergraduate degree and a Master's in Business Administration, as well as earning a credential in public speaking (2014b, pp. 234, 243). At the moment when she receives her MBA diploma, Ramprasad reflects, "*India has given me roots and America has given me wings to fly.* As a child, India had given me a place to belong, a loving family, and a rich heritage. But, as a young woman struggling with depression, it had held me hostage. Eventually, it was America that had blessed me with the freedom and opportunities to discover the power within me to soar in life" (emphasis in original text 2014b, pp. 242–43). Ramprasad views her mental illness not only as the result of a chemical imbalance in the brain or hereditary factors (as mentioned above, her father also suffered from depression, though her parents hid this fact from her), but also as a comprehensible response to the cultural alienation she felt as a young woman growing up in India. In other words, her symptoms, while traumatic, help her understand that adherence to cultural values she intuitively shuns is literally making her ill. When depression stems from cultural alienation, Ramprasad suggests, it can force individuals to fight against oppressive systems and work to create change.

As she becomes stronger, Ramprasad decides to fight alienation and promote systemic change by addressing the conditions which exacerbated her depression in the first place; for, as Raguram et al. remind us, "rather than viewing depression as an essentially *internal* emotional state, it would be prudent to locate it in a much larger, more richly interconnected sociocultural terrain" (2001, p. 33). Born and raised in Bangalore, "the suicide capital of India" (2014b, p. 245), Ramprasad believes that in India, and to a somewhat lesser extent in North America, "people's reluctance to seek mental health services due to stigma is proving to be lethal" (p. 246). After emerging from her depression and finding "the light within," therefore, she became a voice for those experiencing mental illness when she founded ASHA International, a non-profit organization focused on "mental health awareness, hope, and holistic wellness" (2014b, p. 250). Her memoir furthers the work of ASHA, "which literally means 'hope' in Hindi and also in Sanskrit, by sharing her story with others so that they too can find a way to manage mental illness.

Ramprasad's journey also leads her back to where she came from. In most photos on the Internet and in the cover photograph used in *Shadows in the Sun*, Ramprasad chooses to dress in traditional South Asian attire, a departure from her teenage desire to Americanize her appearance. In other words, she identifies herself as a South Asian woman, perhaps to make the point that one can embrace positive aspects of an alienating cultural milieu while also providing impetus for change. As she says in an interview, "when we say *Namaste* in India, it literally means 'the light in me honors the light in you.' And I was blind to my own light for many years" (2014a). Using the metaphor of light versus dark which occurs in the book's title and throughout her text, she writes, "for nearly a decade of my life, as the dark winds of depression blew out the lamp of my mind, body, and soul, I had looked outward, hoping that someone or something could light my darkness away. Yet, in my darkest hour, I discover my *antarjyoti*—the light within. It leads me to a still center that had long eluded me. Amid an ocean of chaos, I discover an island of calm" (2014b, p. 219).

Ramprasad acknowledges the power of some Western technologies, especially talk therapy, to facilitate healing. However, after repeated encounters with Western psychotherapy (which she says helped her), plus antidepressant drugs and electroconvulsive treatments (which did nothing but make her feel worse), Ramprasad realizes that "Western medicine has its limitations. Unlike Eastern modalities of healing that take a holistic approach to treating the mind, body, and spirit, Western medicine is focused on controlling symptoms instead of fostering systems change" (2014b, p. 226). In addition to Western-style talk therapy, then, Ramprasad promotes psychological stability by practicing meditation, postural yoga, and pranayama (monitoring and control of the breath, or the life force). Echoing long-held tenets of yogic philosophy, she also describes how meditation helps her "to become an observer of [her] thoughts and emotions instead of getting entangled in them" (2014b, p. 229).

Applying Carl Elliott's analysis of how alienation can lead to depression and depression can lead to insight, Ramprasad's mental illness eventually forces her to forge a path unique to herself. If, as Jain et al. aver, "achieving a more harmonious balance between the global and the local is one of the most pressing challenges of contemporary Indian psychiatry" (2017, p. 55), Ramprasad's experiences in finding the combination of "Eastern" and "Western" practices which works best for her might point a way forward. Depression narratives, and the depression that begets them, may have value, as they do in Ramprasad's case, because they give people a way to process their unhappiness. Ramprasad's depression was agony while experienced, but provided insights into her entrapment in a set of cultural attitudes she instinctively questioned. By becoming a public face for mental illness, both in India and in America, Ramprasad insists on the right to speak and to be heard, for both herself and for others.

Acknowledgements I would like to thank the editors of this volume, Julie Hollenbach and Robin Alex McDonald, for their helpful insights and suggestions.

References

Ahmed, Sara. 2010. Killing Joy: Feminism and the History of Happiness. *Signs* 35 (3): 571–594.

Almanzar, Santiago, Nirsarg Shah, Suril Vithalani, Sandip Shah, James Squires, Raghu Appusani, and Craig L. Katz. 2014. Knowledge of and Attitudes Toward Clinical Depression Among Health Providers in Gujarat India. *Annals of Global Health* 80 (2): 89–95.

The Bhagavad Gita. 1974. Trans. Swami Nikhilananda. New York: Ramakrishna-Vivekananda Center.

Cvetkovich, Ann. 2012. *Depression: A Public Feeling*. Durham, NC: Duke University Press.

Davis, Lennard J . 2013. *The End of Normal: Identity in a Biocultural Era*. Ann Arbor: University of Michigan Press.

Elliott, Carl. 2003. *Better Than Well: American Medicine Meets the American Dream*. New York: Norton.

———. 2004. Pursued by Happiness and Beaten Senseless: Prozac and the American Dream. In *Prozac as a Way of Life*, eds. Carl Elliott and Tod Chambers, 127–140. Chapel Hill, NC: University of North Carolina Press.

———. 2011. Enhancement Technologies and the Modern Self. *Journal of Medicine and Philosophy* 36: 364–374. https://doi.org/10.1093/jmp/jjr031.

Ghai, Anita. 2009. Disabled Women: An Excluded Agenda of Indian Feminism. In *Rethinking Normalcy: A Disability Studies Reader*, eds. Tanya Titchkosky and Rod Michalko, 296–311. Toronto: Canadian Scholars' Press.

Healy, David. 1997. *The Antidepressant Era*. Cambridge, MA: Harvard University Press.

Jain, Sanjeev, Alok Sarin, Nadja van Ginneken, Pratima Murthy, Christopher Harding and Sudipto Chatterjee. 2017. Psychiatry in India: Historical Roots,

Development as a Discipline and Contemporary Context. In *Mental Health in Asia and the Pacific: Historical and Cultural Perspectives*, eds. Harry Minas and Milton Lewis, 39–57. New York: Springer Science and Business Media. SpringerLink Books—Autoholdings.

Kishore, Jugal, Avni Gupta, Ram Chander Jiloha, and Patrick Bantman. 2011. Myths, Beliefs, and Perceptions about Mental Disorders and Health-seeking Behavior in Delhi India. *Indian Journal of Psychiatry* 53 (4): 324–329.

Kramer, Peter D. 2005. *Against Depression*. New York: Viking.

Kulesza, Magdalena, R. Raguram, and Deepa Rao. 2014. Perceived Mental Health Related Stigma, Gender, and Depressive Symptom Severity in a Psychiatric Facility in South India. *Asian Journal of Psychiatry* 9: 73–77.

Maté, Gabor. 2008. *In the Realm of Hungry Ghosts: Close Encounters with Addiction*. Toronto: Alfred A. Knopf.

Parens, Erik. 2004. Kramer's Anxiety. In *Prozac as a Way of Life*, eds. Carl Elliott and Tod Chambers, 21–32. Chapel Hill, NC: University of North Carolina Press.

Pereira, Bernadette, Gracy Andrew, Sulochana Pednekar, Reshma Pai, Pertti Pelto, and Vikram Patel. 2007. The Explanatory Models of Depression in Low Income Countries: Listening to Women in India. *Journal of Affective Disorders* 102: 209–218.

Raguram, R., Mitchell G. Weiss, Harshad Keval, and S.M. Channabasavanna. 2001. Cultural Dimensions of Clinical Depression in Bangalore India. *Anthropology and Medicine* 8 (1): 31–46.

Raguram, R., Mitchell G. Weiss, S.M. Channabasavanna, and Gerald M. Devins. 1996. Stigma, Depression, and Somatization in South India. *The American Journal of Psychiatry* 153 (8): 1043–1049.

Ramprasad, Gayathri. 2014a. A Conversation with Gayathri Ramprasad. Interview with Rose Caiola. *Rewire Me*, 25 February. https://www.rewireme.com/roses-blog/conversation-gayathri-ramprasad/.

———. 2014b. *Shadows in the Sun: Healing from Depression and Finding the Light Within*. Center City, MN: Hazelden.

Rao, Deepa, Randall Horton, and R. Raguram. 2012. Gender Inequality and Structural Violence among Depressed Women in South India. *Social Psychiatry and Psychiatric Epidemiology* 47: 1967–1975. https://doi.org/10.1007/s00127-012-0504-y.

Robataille, Marie-Claire, and Ishita Chatterjee. 2016. Sex-selective Abortions and Infant Mortality in India: The Role of Parents' Stated Son Preference. *The Journal of Development Studies* 54 (1): 47–56.

Solomon, Andrew. 2001. *The Noonday Demon: An Atlas of Depression*. New York: Scribners.

CHAPTER 13

Toward the Ekstasis of Angels: The Value of Depression in Gwyneth Lewis's Poetry and Memoir

Zoë Brigley Thompson

In "Poetry and Therapy," the psychotherapist J. K. W. Morrice describes the usefulness of poetry for the sufferer of depression and provides a thought-provoking and decorous metaphor. The depressive patient writing poetry is, Morrice explains, "[l]ike the chrysalis … [that] survived the typhoon and, metamorphosed, began to flutter her wings with some surprise, but with a sense of freedom and purpose" (1983, p. 370). Poetry is often invoked as a catalyst for metamorphosis from despair to hope, from desperation to redemption. David Wojahn traces a vein of poetry about depression, noting the "tradition of mad British versifiers" from John Clare onwards, contrasting the British lineage with the American "middle generation"—Sylvia Plath, John Berryman, Robert Lowell et al.—who all "suffered bouts of acute mental anguish resulting in extended hospitalization" (1995, p. 113). Writing through depression,

Z. B. Thompson (✉)
The Ohio State University, Columbus, OH, USA

J. Hollenbach and R. A. McDonald (eds.), *Re/Imagining Depression*,
https://doi.org/10.1007/978-3-030-80554-8_13

however, is far from easy when one aspect of the illness is a "mind-numbing lack of engagement with the world" (Wojahn 1995, p. 115). With this in mind, Wojahn asks: "How do you write poetry at a time when even tying your shoes seems a Herculean labor? And how do you talk to someone about such a frightening predicament?" (p. 115).

These questions are answered, at least in part, by author Gwyneth Lewis (born 1959), who writes about depression in her memoir *Sunbathing in the Rain: A Cheerful Book about Depression* (2006), and her series of poems "Chaotic Angels." The analysis that follows interrogates Lewis's unique view of poetry and depression. For Lewis, the angel is an allegory for epiphanic experiences of the unknown which provide a kind of spiritual grace. This shift in perspective demands *ekstasis*, the act of standing outside of oneself. Drawing on her experience of Zen Buddhist practices and Julia Kristeva's theoretical writings on depression, Lewis uses poetry to transform depression into a luminous gift rather than a debilitating illness, a process she reflects on in her prose. Drawing on Buddhist ideas of "no-self" and Kristeva's description of *ekstasis*, or going beyond oneself, Lewis's angel is a metaphysical being that frames nothingness as epiphanic and redemptive rather than crippling and painful.

The Black Sun

In his essay, "The Dilemma of the Peot" [sic], Don Paterson notes in an aside that, "in a Buddhistic sense the poem teaches you that you're no more than an infinitely malleable, reprogrammable set of habits and characteristics: nothing, in other words" (1996, p. 157). This sense of nothingness is particularly relevant to Lewis, who in her memoir, *Sunbathing in the Rain*, describes the descent into depression as a loss of self. Thinking through the painful lack at the heart of depression, Lewis recalls an etching by Francisco de Goya from the series *Caprichos*, entitled *Que se la llevaron!* (They carried her off). Goya's rendering of a woman carried away by hooded, faceless jailors represents for Lewis "the sensuality of this woman's self-loss" (2006, p. 101). Lewis also associates the picture with the experience of being mugged in New York and, when she writes how "the mugger had taken something of mine," she suggests that the violation of theft triggers a feeling of a greater loss, reminding her of how depression steals any steady sense of identity (2006, p. 109). There is also a benefit to depression since it enables Lewis to write, though "[t]he price of writing was abandoning part of yourself that went, obediently, with your lover, Hades, into the dark" (2006, p. 109). Like Odysseus or other mythical heroes, Lewis must quest down into her own version of Hades to face the unspeakable.

In working out this sense of loss, Lewis draws on psychoanalysis, especially Kristeva's theorising in *Black Sun: Depression and Melancholia* (1989). As William N. Gray summarises, Kristeva views the subject's relationship with the mother as key to depression: "to acquire a subject position in language, in the symbolic order, requires a breaking loose from, a rejection of, the abject, ultimately the mother" (Gray 1996, p. 885). The mother who represents mingling boundaries of the self must be rejected and "[t]he fault which is necessary and ultimately blessed is matricide, for matricide is the condition of the possibility of subjectivity" (Gray 1996, p. 885). The depressive is in a state of mourning for the archaic pre-object or "Thing" which "the depressed person wanders in pursuit of" (Kristeva 1989, pp. 13–14). This Thing is the Black Sun, lifted from Gerard de Nerval's poem, "El Desdichado," translated as "the disinherited," or sometimes as "the alien," a fitting objective correlative for Kristeva's depressive. The Black Sun is intimidating precisely because it represents a loss that can never be assuaged by an ordinary object. In a discouraging reading of the black sun, Kristin Czarnecki suggests that the difficulty in separating from the mother can be deadly for women: "The depressive woman refuses matricide to avoid the tremendous guilt that would accompany it, but in her refusal she harms herself" (Czarnecki 2009, p. 65). In this scenario, the only way to avoid "hatred within" is to express the "hatred and rage" necessary to separate from the mother (Czarnecki 2009, p. 65). Is this misogynist and matricidal scenario the only one possible? Is there no other way out of this bind?

To find another way forward, it might be necessary to graft Kristeva's psychoanalytic theorizing to another kind of practice, as Lewis does. Lewis is intrigued by Kristeva's demand for the depressive to embrace the void of their own melancholy: "Absent from other people's meaning, [...] I owe a supreme, metaphysical lucidity to my depression" (Kristeva 1989, p. 4). Kristeva's black sun obliterates any ordinary sense of self but enables a feeling of metaphysical lucidity. While depressives are "potential exiles" they can also be "intellectuals capable of dazzling, albeit abstract constructions" (Kristeva 1989, p. 64). Using distancing techniques such as allegory, depressives move beyond a conventional selfhood "shifting back and forth from the *disowned meaning*, [...] to the *literal meaning*" (Kristeva 1989, pp. 101–102). Sarah Kay (2013) explains why for Kristeva the use of allegory, symbolic figures and actions that tell us something about human existence, can be extremely important for the depressive. Allegory is a means of "transacting with abyssal absence" and becomes a "hypersign" that is something that "relies on another absent (lost or lacking) sign" (Kay 2013, p. 136). When hovering over a hypertext online, we know that there is more beyond the link in front of us waiting to be discovered, and the hypersign similarly signals a body of knowledge, currents of knowing beyond what is initially seen. Kay gives the example of the expression "Venus rages" because "it stands over and above another sign ('being in love') rather than signifying something directly" (p. 136). Thus Venus suggests "something that is absent and must be sought" and also indicates "the Inexpressibility of the Thing that haunts all language" (p. 137).

This is exactly how the angel works in Lewis's sequence, 'Chaotic Angels,' though the poems are also influenced by Lewis's unique religious practices, and in bringing together her use of Nonconformist Christianity and Zen Buddhism with Kristeva's black sun, Lewis finds a unique perspective lent to her by her knowledge of what it is to be depressed. The religious and spiritual life is very important to Lewis, and she has said that discovering she is "primarily a religious poet" has helped her to understand her depression (1995a, p. 27). She describes this discovery as "a tremendous liberation in relation to language because it means that the values which are most important to me reside not in any one language, but beyond language itself" (p. 27). Part of the significance of Lewis' angel, then, is in its relationship to faith and other unseen, intangible spiritual forces.

Though Lewis is a Nonconformist Christian, she encountered Zen Buddhism through the local Welsh Buddhist community and through lectures from Tibetan Buddhists in Cardiff, all as part of a quest to ease her depression (cf. Lewis 1995b, pp. 81–83). This aspect of her religious practice moves away from the Christian tradition in which, as Dorian Llywelyn describes, there is an obsession with "the disparate spheres of the material and the spiritual, the divine and the human [...] which continually threaten[s] to break down into meaninglessness" (1999, p. 178). Instead, Zen Buddhism embraces meaninglessness, moving beyond a notion of the self as multiple, integral, or unselfconscious, and instead promoting an experience of "no-self" in which focus shifts "from representations of the self to awareness itself" (Engler 2003, p. 65). As Lao Tzu states in the *Tao Te Ching*, only in exile from ordinary ways of thinking and being can one discover the mysteries of life: "Because she has let go of herself, / she is perfectly fulfilled" (Lao Tzu 1999: Chapter 7, lines 8–13). For both Lao Tzu and for Lewis, one can only make progress, feel at ease in the world, and find one's calling by embracing the loss of certainty, attachments and conventional selfhood.

Lewis's practical experience of Zen retreats led her to study its philosophy more closely, because she "no longer wanted to live like a ghost, but to feel the present fully" (2006, p. 88). Lewis explains these ghost-like feelings in terms of what she calls Zen "poverty of spirit," a state of "being so bereft of personality that, even if you wanted to hang yourself you couldn't find a self to hang" (2006, p. 74). Zen practices, however, allow Lewis to turn her lack of selfhood and the emptiness of the void into positive and useful preoccupations: "The Zen meditations which I've learned offer a safe passage through meaninglessness, and prove that confronting it is part of being mentally stable" (2006, p. 136). Lewis has a particular experiential investment in Zen Buddhism and she describes her process of learning with her Japanese Roshi and other spiritual advisors in Cardiff, using the metaphor of "boulders in the river" to describe conscious states of mind that "impede the energy current, but are worn down slowly by the flow, until the Buddha nature eventually breaks through" (p. 88). Only by experiencing the world through the universal mind can higher insights be reached, an achievement that Lewis describes in *Sunbathing in the Rain* through the metaphor of an intuitive "hand" that "without looking, picks up an unrecognisable shape and completes a continent" (2006, p. 176).

The intuitiveness of Zen is made possible by emptiness. Lewis quotes Robert Pirsig's *Zen and the Art of Motorcycle Maintenance* wherein Zen practices such as "koans, deep breathing, sitting still and the like" are described as cultivating a feeling of "stuckness" in the mind which, rather than being a negative state, offers gifts of new perception: "Your mind is empty, you have a 'hollow-flexible' attitude of a 'beginner's mind"' (1974, p. 285). This hollowness in the mind is "not unlike the uses of space—the empty page upon which words can be written, the empty jar into which water can be poured, the empty window through which light can be admitted, and the empty pipe through which water can flow" (Watts 1957, p. 57).

Lewis is self-conscious of her appropriation of Zen rituals as a Westerner, and she criticizes the figure of the "sad Western Buddhist [...] adopting an exotic religion" (Lewis 2006, p. 30). Lewis's grafting of

Zen Buddhist ideas onto Kristeva's theorising of the black sun is valuable, however, as it seeks to avoid the terrible scenario that Kristeva's narrative describes: caught between violent rejection of the mother, matricide even, and violent disgust for one's self. Rather than being stuck in this scenario, the narrators of Lewis's poems give up the desire to be something and seek nothingness instead—even celebrate it. Lewis's allegorical angel steadily attends to the minor, the invisible, and the erased. Lewis's angel is a messenger for hardly visible subjects: angels of dust, of rotting vegetables, of invisible gamma-rays, or of tunes unheard. This is not a message of spiritual perfection but of lost things, and it forces us to ponder what is missing, what is irretrievable.

Angels of Nothingness

The angel is an allegory that works well in the context on Zen Buddhism and Kristeva's notion of *ekstasis*. Angels are significant in poetry; in *The Angel's Corpse*, Paul Colilli compares the angel and poetic logic and links them both to the symbol of the black sun, depression, and the state of being outside oneself (1999, p. 107). Poetry certainly might have something to do with loss, and Lewis suggests that poets are important because "they know more than most about the chaos of life, about living with incompleteness, with hopelessness, [...] the feeling that what you value and cherish most is not valued and cherished by the rest of society" (Lewis 2005b, p. 13). She concludes: "we know what it is to be nobody" (p. 13).

It is impossible to talk about the angel and poetry without mentioning the legacy of Rainer Maria Rilke (1875–1926) and his *Duino Elegies* (1989; first published 1923) which were influenced by the work of Henrich von Kleist. Kleist's model of "a progression of consciousness" created three levels: the unconscious inanimate object (manifested in Rilke via the motif of the puppet), self-conscious man, and the superconscious state of the divine. Kathleen L. Komar explains that the inanimate object and the figure of the divine always have an advantage over human beings, because they "share the ability to participate in a unified existence from which self-conscious human beings are always excluded" (1987, p. 10). For Kleist and Rilke, human existence is predicated on loss, just as Kristeva theorizes in writing about the mourning for the irretrievable Thing.

The angel in Rilke recalls the intimidating Black Sun. In the *First Elegy*, angels are "terrifying," because "beauty is nothing / but the beginning of terror, which we still are just able to endure" (Rilke 1987, pp. 151.7,

151.4–5). The *First Elegy* tells how angels see no "too-sharp distinctions" between the living and the dead, and the *Second Elegy* describes angels as "deadly birds of the soul" existing "behind the stars" whose presence would make "our own heart, beating / higher and higher, [...] beat us to death" (p. 155.83; pp. 157.2, 157.7–9). As Ralph Freedman notes, Rilke's divine being is not a "human Angel," but it is "magnified into an outsized projection of a figure, formed like earthly men and women yet threatening in his infinite range of perception and power" (1998, p. 324). Drawing on biographical detail in Rilke's life, Freedman suggests that "[p]rojecting the figure of the Angel as an original construct of an overpowering and distant consciousness was Rilke's way of breaking through the limits of the private self, confined by the certainty of death" (1998, p. 324). Lewis's journey into *ekstasis* and Zen nothingness overlaps with Rilke's project, but, in contrast to Rilke's angel (described by Freedman as "the perfect, all-powerful figure of God's creation" [1998, p. 324]), Lewis's angels are imperfect, incomplete, and difficult to know.

"Chaotic Angels" is a sequence that comes at the end of Lewis' collection *Keeping Mum* (2003), and is reproduced in her collected works *Chaotic Angels* (2005a). The poems that come before the sequence are a psychiatric detective story investigating a depressive patient, and the answer to the depression is not found through psychiatry but through the angels that are described in a series of poems as an answer to the question posed by the book: how do we survive depression? Drawing on the origins of the word "angel" from the Greek *Angelos* and the Hebrew *Malek*, which both refer to a "messenger," Lewis explains that "the technical term for an unidentified object on a radar screen is 'an angel,' that is a message which we can register, but not fully understand" (Lewis qtd. Rees-Jones 2005, p. 195). The angel is both the messenger and the message. Angels enable those they visit to fulfil an instruction from God and such an exchange recalls the traditional view of angels, as described by Marina Warner, as mediators "between worlds, able to inhabit the intermediate realm because they are themselves intermediaries, messengers from another realm, translating differences of earth and heaven, flesh and spirit" (2006, p. 72).

"Chaotic Angels" is a sonnet sequence that offers representations of unseen forces, self-denial, and the power of selflessness in the face of loss. In "Minimal Angel," Lewis offers a glimpse of what angels might be and to what they might be dedicated:

> The smallest angel of which we're aware.
> is a 'spinning nothing.' Angel of dust,
> angel of stem cells, of pollen grains,
> angel of branches which divide to a blur.
> as they're ready to bud, becoming more.
> than their sum was even an hour before.
> (Lewis 2005a, p. 184.1–6).

Lewis's angel is a contradiction: "a 'spinning nothing'" (p. 184.2). Angels belong to both death and life with allegiances to particles of dust or the waste of human bodies, but also to life-giving stem cells and pollen grains that contain the reproductive gametes of seed plants. The pollen image recalls Rilke's second elegy, which describes the angel as "pollen of flowering godhead" (1987, p. 157.14). As in Rilke, the reproductive qualities of pollen are not simply human but divine too, representing the reproduction of a spiritual message. The finality of the rhyming couplet lends emphasis to the sense of consolation in that fact that the angel is a hypersign standing in for so much more than a physical body: "more/than their sum" (Lewis 2005a, p. 184.5–6).

Lewis's angels also signal qualities that cannot be embodied exactly like wonder, fear, death, life and growth. The volta in the seventh line of "Minimal Angel" marks a change in focus to objects from the practical, modern world:

> Angel of dog smells, angel of stairs,

> … of gardening, marriage. Cherubim.
> of rotting rubbish, of seeing far,
> of rain's paste diamonds after a shower.
> Radiation angels, angels of mud,
> angels of slowing and of changing gear,
> angels of roundabouts, and of being here.
> all say: "You were made for this – prayer."
> (Lewis 2005a, p. 184.7–14).

These angels are seemingly unglamorous and low-key: angels of "dog smells" and "rotting rubbish." The angels emerge too from practical human innovations taken for granted like "stairs," and from more ambiguous discoveries, like radiation, which can harm or help human beings. Not especially good or bad, angels exist in human endeavours, such as the creative act of cultivating a garden, the commitment to another person in marriage, or simply noticing the beauty of nature after a rainstorm. Angels can be part of the everyday lives of human beings; the strong rhyming couplet in the penultimate lines focuses on the mechanics of driving as a metaphor for growth, as the act of changing *gear* translates into a moment in the journey that is *being here*, the rhyme emphasising satisfaction. All of these angels exist in the practical, modern world, rather than being spectacular or startling occurrences. They are stored: in miniscule cells invisible to the human eye, in the slow growth of trees that goes unnoticed, in the low-key, practical existence of the modern world, and in the objects that people cast away from them or ignore. Perhaps if we pay enough attention, there is enough diminutive grace, presence, and vitality to at least distract us from the irretrievable Thing that will never return. Perhaps the depressive might recognize the beauty of the rejected and neglected. Lewis uses the 'Minimal Angel' as an allegory, a hypersign that signals something holy and sacred in these castaway things, in everything.

Angels as Invisible Harmonics

"Pagan Angel" focuses particularly on the invisibility of angels and Lewis concords with Warner's suggestion that the supernatural spirits of the past are still alive but in a different sense to those of the past: "Angels and spectres have changed character, and meaning and impact, but they are visible and powerful through entertainment media in ways that cohere with their past appearances" (2006, p. 335). Lewis's angels are not winged figures or spectacular warriors, but the invisible forces that move through air and bodies:

> You ask me how it is we know.
> God's talking, not us. When even a stone.
> can photograph lilies and, as it falls,
> prove that gravity's no more than speed?
> When loquacious skies call.
> in gamma rays, radio, infra-red,
> and that's if we're not listening at all.
> (Lewis 2005a, p. 180.1–7).

A spiritual problem is posed by the speaker addressing the query of an offstage questioner, and the line-break after "know" signals that this response may not be as straightforward as it initially seems. The stresses falling on "God's" and "us" emphasize that a dialogue is to take place between the divine and the human. The question is how to ascertain the message and presence of God. Polysyllabic words invade the lines with technological and scientific lexicon such as "photograph," "gravity" and "infra-red." These are all powers or forces that work invisibly, yet Lewis asserts that human beings have become blind or deaf to them. Similarly, Lewis expresses wonder at the unseen forces at work in the world such as the processes of geology that create a fossilized imprint of a flower, gravity, and invisible technologies such as gamma, radio and infrared waves. The way in which this discovery is framed, however, registers society's lack of wonder about such discoveries, and faith is difficult in a world in which everything can be explained. As a remedy for this failure, Lewis looks to the human body:

> The heart's a chamber whose broody dead.
> stage pagan rituals. Wind blows.
> across stone lintels, making a tune.
> about absent bodies.
> You ask me again:
> "Where's the angel acoustic?".
> My dear, the curlew. The quickening rain.
> (Lewis 2005a, pp. 180.8–14).

The first line of this section marks a volta as the logic moves from considering human beings' disbelief to examination of the human interior. The opening line is rhythmic and emphatic, the content accentuating the message that the heart is much more than a mechanical organ. The heart, inhabited by dead people, is a space in which improbable or unbelievable things could occur. "[P]agan rituals" are performed in the heart, recalling sub-cultures on the margins of European Christianity. Lewis envisions wind blowing through the chamber of the heart, blustering around the lintels, those stone slabs that discharge the weight of the structure above. The breeze creates a music "about absent bodies," an ambiguous phrase that offers two meanings; either the "tune" is on the theme of absent bodies, or the preposition, "about," describes the wind moving around the location of the heart and between the "absent bodies" of the dead. In either case, the tune emerges from nothingness. Lewis uses an Aeolian harp, that Romantic symbol for giving up the self to some other power, to discover an "angel acoustic." Lewis can only describe this acoustic obliquely, gesturing to the everyday sounds of nature: birdsong and rainfall. The curlew is a wading bird renowned for its musical cry, but there is also the "curlew sign," a notation in musical score. In this context, the curlew represents the emptiness of the sign that enables human beings to communicate, while the rain might represent celestial grace as it does in so many religious narratives and mythologies. The rhyme between "again" and "rain" emphasizes the rain as a reoccurrence of God's presence in the world and the "Pagan Angel" as hypersign gestures towards the holy and answers the disbelief of the first part of the sonnet.

Belief and disbelief reoccur in the "Chaotic Angels" sonnet sequence, and often the invisible force of the divine can only make its presence felt through music or sound. In *Phantasmagoria*, Marina Warner describes the initial amazement in the nineteenth century at "the possibility of previously undetected acoustic phenomena" (2006, p. 258). Warner describes the sense of wonder at the fact that, "that harmonic maps hummed beyond the reach of human senses, and that the universe was vibrating with imperceptible forces" (p. 258). Music and the imperceptible are also significant in Christian theology. For example, when Simone Weil writes about faith, she uses the metaphor of music: listening to God is like "When we listen to Bach or to a Gregorian melody, all the faculties of the soul become tense and silent in order to apprehend this thing of perfect beauty" (Weil 1947, p. 129). For Weil and Lewis, faith rests upon the act of listening and maintaining silence. Lewis describes music as "an angelic force at the centre of current world turmoil," and she situates music in opposition to violence (2002,p. 81).

"Fire Angel" uses a similar metaphor when Lewis suggests that "it's music that holds up this church" (2005a, p. 182.1). Expanding the metaphor, Lewis imagines further fortifications such as "chromatic buttresses" and "a spandrel wall/ of finest vibrato" (2005a, p. 182.2–3). The term, "chromatic," is used in music to describe notes absent from the scale of the key of a particular passage (i.e. non-diatonic notes). Meanwhile the spandrel wall that supports an arch is made not from bricks but from the singing technique, vibrato, a fluctuation of pitch, intensity, and timbre. Far from being sturdy fortifications, these supports are off-key and insubstantial. Indeed, the church spire "narrows to nothing on its rising scale, / leaning the weathercock to turn at will / prompted by any weathery whim" (2005a, p. 182.4–6). The spire, however, directs the parishioners to the weathercock, which like the heart that becomes an Aeolian harp in "Pagan Angel," is moved by the invisible force of the wind. "Fire Angel" and "Pagan Angel" both gesture in allegorical terms to what is beyond human perception, and in both poems, this offers a kind of consolation.

Angels of Death

In opposition with music, Lewis depicts fire. Music is sometimes the victor; the first half of "Fire Angel" concludes with the lines: "Melody, for once, has overcome fire" (2005a, p. 182.7). The volta occurs, however, when Lewis states: "But I've seen different" (p. 182.8). The poem shifts to Acco, an ancient city mentioned in the Old Testament as part of a parcel of land belonging to the Sheret of Asher (cf. Judges 1.31). Situated in modern-day Israel, Acco has historically always been a site of contest fought over by the Egyptians, Syrians and Chinese. By the thirteenth century, French and English crusaders had gained control of the city and constructed a vast network of underground passages beneath the city. In the second half of "Fire Angel," Lewis describes entering this secret complex following a boy "who lit up plastic-bottle flares / and guided me, nervous, underground" (p. 182.9–10). The "plastic-bottle flares" situate the experience firmly in the modern day, yet the language moves from the throwaway materials of the contemporary moment "into flickering vaults, a garrison / built by crusaders, remembered in flame" (p. 182.13–14). On a visual level, the vaults might be "flickering" as the subjects view them by candlelight, yet there is also a feeling that the garrison, a body of troops to protect a town, is not human at all, but embodied by fire like the Old Testament angels, for example in Exodus 3:2, when the Angel of the Lord appears to Moses in the form of a burning bush. This kind of angel is associated in Lewis's poem with the violence and warfare of Acco. The flame is seductive, yet Lewis's philosophy of the angel rejects the punitive Old Testament model as the sonnet comes to an end.

Another poem, "Tarot Angel," considers avenging angels in Revelations which celebrate the linguistic division of humankind (cf. Revelation 14.8). Lewis suggests human mistrust and division emerges from fear "of the Death card and the Hanging Man / though what they signify is far from clear" (p. 181.6–7). In the Tarot pack, the symbol of Death might represents a literal death or metaphorical one, while the symbol of the Hanging Man has its origins in Germanic mythology: the story of Odin, who in a quest of self-sacrifice for the gift of wisdom, hung himself on the cosmic tree to learn the secrets of the runes. Both symbols dictate a loss of selfhood, and they recall the act of slipping into the void.

"Tarot Angel" traces a journey towards embracing the void, and after the volta half-way through the poem, it moves from the difficulties of linguistic difference to praise the seemingly impossible belief in immortality.

> Who says this is folly? It might come true.
> Step over the cliff with me, the Fool,
> take a chance on changing. Die every day.
> as if you were living and that you knew.
> that broad roads score the blazing sky.
> (Lewis 2005a, p. 181.10–14).

In spite of uncertainty, Lewis's invitation (in the second line) to believe that death itself is a hypersign concealing unfathomable depths is intriguing. The emphasis that falls on the word "cliff" reveals that this poem is situated on the edge of conventional thinking. The broken rhythm highlights the uncertainty of faith and its difficulty, yet the final line with its three long stresses on "broad roads score" lingers over the possibilities of faith. Also the half-rhyme between "day" and "sky" focuses on the possibilities and vastness of time and space. Conveying a message of hope, the "Tarot Angel" contrasts with the Biblical angel of Revelations that celebrates human mistrust and division. To reach this state, however, means opening up to the prospect of death as a hypersign, and by celebrating nothingness, peace and grace can be found.

The final poem in the sequence, "Christ as an Angel of the Will of God" dwells on this message going beyond even "our need for angels" cultivating a relationship with the divine beyond the need for allegorical mediators, or by becoming the mediator oneself (Lewis 2005a, p. 191.2). Lewis has written that Christ can appear in any kind of everyday setting: "I think of Christ as anything or anyone who shows up the nature of God, like dust in a stream of sunlight" (Lewis qtd. Rees-Jones 2005, p. 195). Lewis describes how it is possible to glimpse the divine in everyday life, and to express this, Lewis creates complex metaphors, such as the possibility of "calculat[ing] the logarithms of grace / to easy solutions in our sleep" (Lewis 2005a, p. 191.5–6). It is significant that Lewis imagines a condition of unconsciousness, sleep, as the best possible state in which to discover the divine, recalling Weil's comment that "Grace fills empty spaces but it can only enter where there is a void to receive it, and it is grace itself that makes this void" (1947,p. 10).

How might Lewis discover a new generative poetics and the kind of decreation that Weil recommends? Like the early Christian ascetics, or the Buddhist sects of wandering asceticism, Lewis strips away her selfhood and as she explains in interview, what she recommends losing are "ideas about yourself [...] ideas about what poetry is about, what you're about, as well as others' ideas about you" (2005b, p. 12). As Anne Carson states, the act of decreation as defined by Weil is "an undoing of the creature in us—that creature enclosed in self and defined by self," yet the path to such decreation is difficult since, "to undo self one must move through self, to the very inside of its definition" (2006, p. 179). Might it be possible to become aware of ourselves as hypersigns, or at least to understand ourselves as containing space for the unfathomable and unknowable?

Moving through and unravelling her selfhood, Lewis discovers what is beyond simple and conventional identity: nothingness. The angel emerges from the frustrated language of depression to conjure *ekstasis* where the allegory is a powerful antidote to loss. What finally emerges is a more complicated understanding of how to overcome despair, depression, profound loss. This project becomes then what Kristeva describes as "the admirable face of loss, transforming it in order to make it live" (1989, p. 99). Lewis escapes the unbearable scenario of always seeking the irretrievable Thing, and her angel allegories work as hypersigns to suggest the possibility of things unseen and unspoken connected to the sacred. One reward, of depression according to Lewis' reading of Kristeva, is the poetic gift, since depression, like poetry, is "beyond words, beyond sense" (Lewis 2006, p. 42). The idea of the "beyond" is emphasized in Kristeva as a space of *ekstasis* or being beyond oneself, where the aesthetic is a powerful antidote to loss: "In the place of death and so as not to die of the other's death, I bring forth—or at least I rate highly—an artifice, an ideal, a 'beyond' that my psyche produces in order to take up a position outside itself—*ek-stasis*" (1989, p. 99). Poetry and the play of language offer the possibility of sublimating loss, and this is the compensation of depression's void as it enables a new and complex vision. Using *Black Sun* and Zen Buddhist practices promoting ideas of nothingness, Lewis describes the painful process of being in the thralls of depression, but ultimately, Lewis concludes that her feelings of nothingness may allow her to achieve a metaphysical state.

References

Carson, Anne. 2006. *Decreation: Poetry, Essays, Opera*. London: Jonathan Cape.

Colilli, Paul. 1999. *The Angel's Corpse*. Basingstoke: Macmillan.

Czarnecki, Kristin. 2009. "Yes, It Can Be Sad, Sun in the Afternoon": Kristevan Depression in Jean Rhys's *Good Morning Midnight*. *Journal of Modern Literature* 32 (3): 63–82.

Engler, Jack. 2003. Being Somebody and Being Nobody: A Re-examination of the Understanding of Self in Psychoanalysis and Buddhism. In *Psychoanalysis and Buddhism: An Unfolding Dialogue*, ed. Jeremy D. Safran, 35–79. Boston, MA: Wisdom Publications.

Freedman, Ralph. 1998. *Life of a Poet: Rainer Maria Rilke*. Evanston, IL: Northwestern University Press.

Gray, William N. 1996. George Macdonald, Julia Kristeva, and the Black Sun. *Studies in English Literature, 1500–1900* 36 (4): 877–893.

Gray, Katherine. 2005. Gwyneth Lewis in America. *New Welsh Review* 70: 8–13.

Gregson, Ian. 2005. Negotiations. *Planet: The Welsh Internationalist* 173: 50–56.

Kay, Sarah. 2013. Allegory and Melancholy in Luce Irigaray, Julia Kristeva, and Christine de Pizan. *Textet: Studies in Comparative Literature* 70: 125–140.

Komar, Kathleen L. 1987. *Transcending Angels: Rainer Maria Rilke's Duino Elegies*. Lincoln, NE: University of Nebraska Press.

Kristeva, Julia. 1989. *Black Sun: Depression and Melancholia*. Trans. Leon S. Roudiez. New York: Columbia University Press.

Lewis, Gwyneth. 1995a. Gwyneth Lewis Talks to Richard Poole. *Poetry Wales* 31 (2): 24–29.

———. 1995b. On Writing Poetry in Two Languages. *Modern Poetry in Translation* 7: 80–83.

———. 1998. Tenuous and Precarious: The Comic Muse. *Poetry Review* 88 (3): 17–19.

———. 2000. Whose Coat Is that Jacket? Whose Hat Is that Cap? In *Strong Words: Modern Poets on Modern Poetry*, eds. W.N. Herbert and Matthew Hollis, 265–269. Tarset, ND: Bloodaxe.

———. 2002. Chaotic Angels: A Programme Note. In *The City Of London Festival Programme 2002*. London: City of London Festival.

———. 2005a. *Chaotic Angels: Poems in English*. Tarset, ND: Bloodaxe.

———. 2005b. Gwyneth Lewis in America. Interview by Kathryn Gray. *New Welsh Review* 70: 8–13.

———. 2006. *Sunbathing in the Rain: A Cheerful Book about Depression*. London: Harper Perennial.

———. 2008. Criss-Crossings: Literary Adventures on Irish and Welsh Shores. *Poetry Review* 98 (3): 54–72.

Llywelyn, Dorian. 1999. Cardiff: University of Wales Press.

Morrice, J.K.W. 1983. Poetry as Therapy. *British Journal of Medical Psychology* 56: 367–370.

Paterson, Don. 1996. The Dilemma of the Peot [sic]. In *How Poets Work*, ed. Tony Curtis, 155–172. Bridgend: Seren.

Pirsig, Robert. 1974/1999. *Zen and the Art of Motorcycle Maintenance: An Enquiry into Values*. London: Vintage

Rees-Jones, Deryn. 2005. *Consorting With Angels: Essays on Modern Women Poets*. Tarset, ND: Bloodaxe.

Rilke, Rainer Maria. 1987. *The Selected Poetry of Rainer Maria Rilke*, ed. Stephen Mitchell and trans. Stephen Mitchell. London: Picador.

Thompson, Zoe Brigley. 2007. Personal communication. 3 April 2007.

Tzu, Lao. 1999. *Tao Te Ching*, trans. Stephen Mitchell. London: Frances Lincoln.

Warner, Marina. 2006. *Phantasmagoria: Spirit Visions, Metaphors and Media into the Twenty-First Century*. Oxford: Oxford University Press.

Watts, Alan W. 1957. *The Way of Zen*. London: Penguin.

Weil, Simone. 1947/2002. *Gravity and Grace*, trans. Emma Crawford and Mario von der Ruhr. London: Routledge.

Wojahn, David. 1995. The State You Are Entering: Depression and Contemporary Poetry. *New England Review* 17 (1): 110–123.

CHAPTER 14

Bird Says the Sound of Rewind

Hamish Ballantyne and Fan Wu

SPORE PRINTS

fowl called fucking
Oldsquaw for its scream
That ~~day~~ a jam ~~day~~ ~~new~~ lang syne
pierre friend of
the pianow and prospects
for gold   ~~chillo~~
  chillo sliced ~~through~~
up the ~~zinging~~ particulate
      freeze

* * *

H. Ballantyne
Terrace, BC, Canada

F. Wu (✉)
Queen's University, Kingston, ON, Canada

J. Hollenbach and R. A. McDonald (eds.), *Re/Imagining Depression*,
https://doi.org/10.1007/978-3-030-80554-8_14

~~distinctive~~ ~~no~~
~~whiteout~~ ~~blank~~ ~~stickers~~
not
the whale nor
~~wing of~~ the yuletide psychotic
distinctive no—
the ~~real~~ whale free
willy was ~~poisoned~~
~~off~~ ~~near~~
~~in the Iceland~~

* * *

~~fish truckload~~
Trucked with poison
Creeps
Downseas

* * *

all at
christmas ~~blue light~~ ~~grubby~~ sky falls ~~over~~ all
over the mountains

christmas ducks
the island tied up off there

* * *

mountains of the coast with
skies on
a species ~~thing~~
is a patchup
reckoning—
pink ink of the
baikal teal era

~~lake pond swamp~~
Unravelling
~~Strands~~

* * *

all-night sun haunt in the room
mere pebbles away the tracks
~~lurching~~ ~~a larch~~
Larch zing zing
zing zing
snowflake translation (comes
closer to quiet than
any train
slamming away

* * *

warpen ol larch
springtide ~~warmupburble~~
~~forgotten~~ studying
postures ~~trick knee~~
THEY haven't come
by in a
while
Speak to me of lake Baikal

* * *

don't seem
to GET it he
ALWAYS made a
Hello
Soaked my oils

His lake
baikal oilskins
—clippings for the
monster's scrapbook

* * *

fog clambers down
the acre   drip
drip   spore print i'm
lonesome
Mulling rogue
ways of the ~~adults~~ applemen
~~fruit crate~~
mulling a
mosey somewhere

* * *

one vulture can
anthrax an ox herd
under
~~no oxen here~~
~~steady~~
~~breathing moo up~~
Shove ~~the~~ beef in the
~~good~~ wine   if I go
the ~~whole~~ the
adults
must also
go

These days the body is a series of stoppages, a wound between the thrum & shudder, *warpen ol larch* lurch along the tracks that the unnameable have trod, the abject ideals of lossy life. The psychic wound is secondary to the physical wound: when our flesh is ill our energies spill back into the body to heal it; the mind tends to the body before it can attend to either its immaterial neuroses or worldly anxieties. In illness, the libido—normally a roaming thing that searches for things to latch onto—never garners enough energy to project itself into an outer world or other life; anhedonia anesthetizes us from feeling our body, all our nurture turned inward. Yet illness and sadness form their own particular closed loop that afflicts the mind. Sealed in a body broken down, what I mourn is the possibility of mourning, of a first-order sadness that now eludes me. Nauseous and stooped over I feel not the ache of missing those I love, but the ache of the inaccessibility of even that missing, which would at least grant me the favour of being felt. Anhedonia grows until it forecloses: no future, no past: it looms over you as absolute substance. Terror idea! that once love has been overtaken, it can never be reeled back into the body to which it once belonged. *I'm lonesome Mulling rogue.*

Does the individual body, by falling apart, sense the extinction of the species it belongs to, like one of those giant Chinese bowls that would drop a bronze berry in a bronze frog's mouth at the first sign of an encroaching earthquake? Avernus is the mythological gate to hell before which birds fall dead. What is it in the bird—the vulture and the duck and of course canary—that make it such a symbol for premonition, the human's near future foretold by these creature's present deaths? We envy their freedom, and so we turn them into the symbols of a morbid sensitivity synonymous with mortality, into the sacrifices we make at the coal mine's mouth in order that we might live. A spore print is the outline of a fungus pressed down onto paper. It is a different impression of what will survive us. Extinction brings me the giddy joy of the possibility of partaking in the same blanket death as everyone I love, everyone I hate. Such an insulated fantasy of extinction exists mostly to counteract the probability that the rich will live on as the poor survive. *A species thing is a patch up reckoning.*

Illness severs you from a form of life whose attachments you once relied upon. I wake, my crushes dimmed out, my desire lines snuffed. The fantasy of playing a witness at your own funeral is rendered in glorious technicolour. Cataplexy makes the social cut out, a television badly wired. Hanging out indiscernible from spazzing out. How many ways can I use the word *body* before it's exhausted, the body mesmerized by a new symptom every day, the body *trucked with poison creeps downseas?* Limbs askew, *clippings for the monster's scrapbook*, a stochastic sickness that randomizes the self's obstructions against itself. Then again, the body's glitches and slips are mostly unknown to others, save the occasional slurred sentence stuttered panic-stricken by my leaden tongue. Deleuze revelled in the slowness that his sick body brought him, allaying the ceaseless flow of capitalist time whose productivity-orientation obliterates daily perception (Boutang 1996). And an efficient way to excuse himself from life's unnecessaries: it suited him just fine to be excluded from the circuit of academic meet and greets, from the exhausting thoughtlessness of travel, from the chores of sociality. Listening to Lana Del Rey on my sickbed: *God bless America*, and the reprieve my body grants me in moments of grace. To one day be able to see my illness as a proliferation of selves, temporalities, perspectives within myself: this is the frame upon my illness toward which I strive; not to recuperate myself unto health, but rather to launch my illness unto sublimity.

specially dark a mind
casts the line after
association
~~Longing~~
invented a mountain
range—the specifics
of a time spent
there   waking
heating coffee
a video life
there   in the sights
of a morning thing

* * *

Can you ~~believe~~
believe one
signal light gone dead
threes
bleep up the remains
of a tempo

not so dark
~~dark and there~~

~~moon spoils~~
if not for the fat moon the
bay is
the breath of a whale

* * *

EARTHQUAKE
is it
the dirt
licker (disintegrates)
parafriend
storied in the clink

this old body never
strays from the can

DREAM a heron or owl
what's of importance
here is form
   at night fringed
with glimmers
~~ie Glowstickperimeter~~
—now it's socked in here   how
to write about this stuff when
im honest don't want
   to anymore
I have eaten
well of late   outside the house there
was an owl
waiting
for us to smoke
up

* * *

NOTES: FROM THE TELLY
the freedom to
   follow totally a
feeling
migration
always stands in for
freedom
follows the logic of
  freedom as need
at the instant of
emoting
   NOTES FROM A BOOK
   ~~claw-sighted~~
Bernadette glares at
   some mountain (of the
mind: and hazards a
   beer
  yearns for
blues grosbeak

    agnes
varda clutches the forms of
    migrants   picking
the fields
    a varda a grosbeak
    assembled for sunflowers
    ~~hook sighted~~

The bird landscapes of Hamish Ballantyne are incidental, nearly without incident except the minor event of each line's own life. The poem stitches actuality and wish-projections and mind-muttered annoyances with the capacity of consciousness to blend such distinctions away. He watches Bernadette (Mayer) replicate his own motions: *Bernadette glares at/some mountain (of the/mind: and hazards a/beer.* As though she reached into the panorama of those imagined mountains to draw, from its muddy streams and inlets, a beer. The poem realizes the continuity of perception by herding world into the Virtual; thought is action as action becomes thought. I keep coming back to the DREAM verse, how it's glutted with a boyish resistance, the tantrum-tinged *don't wanna* interrupting the abstractions of a woodland night. I hear the line *Im honest dont want* in its autonomy—plainly, and with open palms, no desire for this, no desire of any kind—perhaps it's been whetted to a nub under the satiation of *I have eaten/well of late*, perhaps too well to keep wanting more. But the owl, who proffers a prophetic figuration of the landscape's fringe and glimmer, contradicts the narrator's wantlessness with its Minervan waiting, patient in its predatory way. (What does it cost for us to distinguish DREAM from its obscure obverse?) And the next action of a life begins, a blaze, a break.

Health returns to me on the coattails of its reluctance. In the vireo's eye, in the dangling forests of Hypnos, in the hush of another callous dawn. *Specially dark a mind/casts the line after/association/Longing*. The longing for health is a longing for association, yes the social, *parafriends* in proximity; but also for language to come back into the openness of association, so each word may glint again shadowy with surprises, and each line again contain a universe.

In his poem "Spelt from Sibyl's Leaves", Gerard Manley Hopkins's apocalyptic image of depression is "a rack / Where, selfwrung, selfstrung, sheathe- and shelterless, thóughts agaínst thoughts ín groans grínd," the mind contracted into a pinhole-sized machine, too small to let barely any world in (Hopkins 1964). For Hopkins, the ecstasy of the world—the infinite play of its variability—is annihilated by the profundity of self-doubt, which turns world into war. What Hopkins casts as self-doubt I feel as hypochondria, the groan of thought against body, thought interpreting then living its own interpretation of the body as sickness. In my bursts of health I leave my body forgotten. The very fact that the body appears on the scene of thought means something has failed. The line *This old body/never strays from the can* I read in hope, even as I dream of a body that never strays from the *must*—that exists simply in its own necessity, never to trespass its proper role of total silence.

the last time you knew
anyone—searching
   the ground for your
keys and
everyone wants to catch your
eye   ~~coming~~
~~coming / going~~

* * *

vireo makes the sound of
rewind   coming back to
     oneself (vireo
a new world

     species—coming to health
etc.~~faceof this~~
   miniature

     dove glitches
by a green
   pool

* * *

~~addendum~~
~~makeup words~~
     the funeral devours
     relief on waking
the dream a palm with a long
line of terror   in
the end   dressed many times
   for the same
          funeral

     at
times I looked
   I was   older than

myself now~~—country~~
~~home~~
        yellows
                news
      in the evening ~~driveway~~
my home   at
         times   younger
And younger without
         missive
but mum
barefoot

~~sidewalk~~

sidewalk
    ~~days of piling~~
still   ~~in the car~~
    listened to country
in the car
three boys as kids ~~peering~~
       ~~brother~~

                fruit tree
Unsure in photos

get dressed
get in the car

"I've been spending some fairly bad days preoccupied with my health, with that feverishness returning as it did two months ago. I think I will have to go for an X-ray today. Health is stupid. It is essential and yet we can only talk about it in a dull way. And others also are very bad at talking about it to us. For me, it has been four years and I am still not resigned to being sick" (Barthes 2018, p. 59). This is what Barthes writes to his beloved Robert David from the confines of the sanatorium. For him, one's relationship to health is caught between negative and negative: either one resists, or one resigns. One day the *sound of rewind* will play me back into who I was, not so withdrawn into my own flesh, simply exhausted in the ordinary way. No, never will there be a *coming back to oneself*; the body is a new world and so why not take comfort in the new world's reconstitution of itself into stark novelty, moment by moment? Between the fantasy of coming back and the resignation of unshakeable illness are crevices for nostalgia to sustain me, *three boys as kids/fruit tree/get dressed/get in the car*. Get me

back to California's
Polly-Anna ice
        cream song   hella
hand-in-hand with grandpa
                in beach house in
all but tatters

"'

Every time I get a slight headache or felt a slight ache or pain in my body, I prayed I wasn't dying, so that I could see you again. It is on behalf of you that I will not die. It is only love that reproduces, in its staggering limping in its weakness, the sense of life as worthy of life. Last week I learned the word *cuffing*: that is the desire to have one body to hold during winter and to give to that body the whole power of the hearth, your hearth my heart to his touch turns a massive leech who dreams that what was sickness turns terminal, fever dream on fever dream of funeral and all those he called *friend* once weeping at the grave, brick upon brick the soil of love poured over his body undone body, both sickness and love implying full systematic failure, *my self now the yellowed news*, what else to call the name of our lying beside each other arm-in-arm, how else cull from the overabundant banquet of the Now a form of life worthy of the name unlisp-ed, could love then be the remaking of your fragility in space by mine in rhythm, the body that quakes, the body that quivers, the body that acquiesces to the mouth that pukes, the mouth that speaks, the mouth that shivers? For into a blank manner you asked me to do what I cannot do. All the shame in me stopped against my tongue.

or prefer dying
than collect what
you forgot
in someone's house——w/o even going over—like a pretext—viz. lie—but
will it
be worth it— and what
precisely did I leave

the days are unbearable

sleepwalking "the plates
smashed all
over the ground"
incredible dismay (was a cow
boy quick
hand among the dishes—

* * *

mi mango mi chloro
ese queridísimo mes
de julio
drunk scourges et all
the lily shoots on
that block and after upon
the table fucked

* * *

returning not like green spring
—you are the camera
that devoured my soul
and give me shitty
picture like
shitty wine + wafer thank
GOD for FIRE to burn
all photographs
(you can never go back so
long
as you
can be gone back to

* * *

as usual am writing
w/o permission but she
will never know/read/see/hear/care
was under the hum
of trees and I heard
her crunching thru the brush
And later knew I didn't
care when I saw
those trees
growing in the goalmouth
of my childhood—and an unknown
number now means only SCAM, no it is a breeze, warm, unknown
only since rupture, a sea-breeze from prior optimism
(plant rosemary flowers stay
on in sea-breeze
no it is a SCAM no notion other
in my redcurrant
heart

* * *

an embroidered
tablecloth don't
forget the sad
knight's discourse on the hoary
thread side
flowers on the tablecloth
flowers on the trees
dearth of bees
of beers
to fuck and fuck and drink

* * *

lo colourful
reef
blue waters
everyone
utterly crazy

criminals
driven salt wild
tooth stays
in first fruit
you ate in a while
land! loss!
lo bright
reef

* * *

for you fan i want
to be hungover in a cascade
of dust maybe partially
unwelcome in your thoughtful
hours   go about
the work of helping
you welcome me—conjure
a squalid meal
make a tomato
        joke call the beautiful
ghost that lives
in tweaky dance
steps

* * *

NATALIE as a girl
would sleepwalk into the
wall endlessly at the edge
of a videogame world
fretting—where's my apple

after months without speaking
a language first thing
to go are synonyms

        gift lonely
    murmur

And then Coronavirus hits, changing the terms of *bird* and *depression* both.

And though it was a year ago that you wrote those last verses, the pungency of our fantasy of being-together only now under pandemic makes itself truly felt. J Hamish, you would never be unwelcome in thoughtful hours because your life around me is by itself thought, burning thought, thought immune to inertia. Would that we could start the mornings swooning on cigarettes and juice to spill into afternoon stomach aches then wreck our tiny minds on some out-of-frame sadness that rounds our perfect ephemeral domesticity, two boys for whom everything beyond survival feels like drag.

After months without speaking/a language first thing/to go are synonyms. Our old form of life has been laid bare. It's only been weeks, but February seems like historical fiction now. A language without synonyms is boiled down to its essentials; there's no more substitution, no more choice. But, choiceless, every moment is narrowed into emergency precision, and we stand with existential lucidity over the thinness of our lives.

It's a thinness, not bereft of richness, of *gift lonely/murmur*, the susurrations of finally the urgency of communitarian care. Spirit takes the stage hand-in-hand with pragmatism and prophetic talk is rekindled as we begin to forge new futures. The gifts are lonely because we slip them under the doors of our quarantined friends (backlash of skin hunger and horniness), but a sharper vision of love takes to voice as a bird'd take to wing. It begins as a murmur.

How does it end? How does it feel to be trapped inside of the world-historical? Suddenly, at least as long as I'm relatively healthy under a pandemic, there's no room for depression; rather, depression transmogrifies into a mixture of exhilaration and vigilance. We grieve what we'd been taking for granted, which is the ordinariness of daily life, where even its chaos could be counted on. At the same time we grasp in hope at life otherwise than it was, because the ordinary "back then" was already corrupted by—to use a bloated signifier—Capitalist consumption. (Yet we are sharply aware that the ones who craft world history come from a class of people who have the capacity to register this state of emergency as distinct from a state of stability; who aren't simply always, by the dynamics of Capitalist exploitation, plunged into emergency).

You can never go back so long as you can be gone back to. I love you, and my tentative waiting upon the mend of our physical distance takes this love's form.

most dark in my quarter
stalking in my longpants I play
heron
chancer on the tracks of a cuppa

chances, chances
that a boat's shadow traps the clam
seafloor
seafloor
chanting meteor
slow as the thought
takes to roll the
length of a hammock
doubling back
on myself
someone to see

References

Barthes, Roland. 2018. *Album: Unpublished Correspondences & Texts*. New York: Columbia University Press.

Boutang, Pierre-André. 1996. *L'Abécédaire de Gilles Deleuze*. France.

Hopkins, Gerard Manley. 1964. Spelt from Sibyl's Leaves. *Poems and Prose*. Ed. W.H. Gardner. London: Penguin.

CHAPTER 15

The Present is What We Are Doing Together

Feel Tank Chicago

The history of the present moment is (mostly) about not being able to keep up with, or track of, the barrage of incidents that happen in times when there is a looming social, political, and personal threat. The present is being hesitant to speak, do, make, love, but still and nonetheless being willing to speak, do, make, love. It presents itself in non-sequiturs, riffs, the rehearsal of comebacks and retorts. When charted it looks like a zigzag, pointing in one thought and direction then moving (too quickly) to another, as Erykah Badu sings "on and on and on and on" in "my cypher keeps moving like a rolling stone" (Badu 1997).

There are personal rants, some heard for the first time, finally finding a place outside of the head. It is (mostly) about coming to the table where we meet and stalling the event. Because if there is anything we learn from the history of the present moment, it is that the event will be stalled.

The event, the one that (mostly) matters in the present, is stalling the other historical events that our beleaguered raced, gendered, classed, and ill bodies need to make sense of, and maybe even expurgate, before we can get to the next idea. We desire an outcome: the opaque mass of reasons

F. T. Chicago (✉)
Chicago, IL, USA
e-mail: mpatte@artic.edu

J. Hollenbach and R. A. McDonald (eds.), *Re/Imagining Depression*,
https://doi.org/10.1007/978-3-030-80554-8_15

why we don't participate, when non-participation is not an option. We're dying to be on the same page, queasy about what's next.

But what is the event of the present, toggling between Badu to Badiou? Badiou argues that the event is a radical break with the reproduction of what's ongoing. He doesn't think it's a moment of hesitation and overcoming hesitation. He doesn't think it involves repressing the vital forces. He thinks the event initiates the decomposition of the world. It "extracts from a time the possibility of an other time" (Badiou 2007, p. 39). It's not freedom from and freedom for: it creates a crisis that opens new historical formations to the imaginary and praxis.

If we are stalled out in the present we are unmaking and making together, rather than thinking of a blockage as a premonition of revolution, a revolutionary rumble the scanners are picking up, Badiou helps us see the yellow light, at least. The slowdown command. Can we appreciate our breath?

But if the future requires the destruction of the present in a radical cut, what does the destruction of continuity feel like? This is where we resist Badiou: the present is not a cut; it's an effect of an action, a sketching of the map of what we hold together, a convergence of forces, a shift from the compulsive reproduction that lets us celebrate just getting through things (a mud pie party where we feel out forms of the otherwise, new substances of copresence).

It may be that we need each other's help to turn the brain fog into an atmosphere we can all take in, move through, leap from.

Stalled tactics. The decades-long tantrum. Marking time since the Great Recession. Never being able to reach the present. Catching up with ourselves. The hamster on the wheel, or the ever-on-the-move Sweetback in Melvin Van Peebles' hard-to-watch film (Van Peebles 1971). Bernie's urgency, in retrospect. They wear themselves out trying to stop.

Never being able to reach the present is exhausting. The only constant is the delusion that it has finally arrived, that one has finally caught up. But really one is caught up, entangled, even stuck in histories—nearly all of which are too unresolved to fit nicely into the past.

When you improvise the present it comes—in a burst or very subtly, short term usually. It is synonymous with being free, like in the way that Black people try to feel free for a brief duration, before a national or personal crisis occurs. Then the present stops and the past comes rushing in. And the fatigue comes rolling in: it's tiring to wait for another encounter with the present. Instead, you take in or embrace the exhaustion that represents the not-present; own it. Make something of it. Consider what projects and objects can be made with its material. This is the riddle of "getting by," making and producing in spite of exhaustion. The emphasis is not on a lack of resources. It's about lack of time in the present because that's where life is situated.

* * *

By now you know that we regard the present as different things. Some of us think it's a thing, some of us think it's a political concept rooted in affect and analysis. The present is what we are doing together: a space in (some version of) common: a desire to generalize together (Some of what follows is cut, pasted, rearranged).

A present defined by the desire for something to be over. The present refreshed. Caught in the act; in the fullness of a different now. Anxiety and the future. Dating things to kill them. "That was then, this is now." Depression as a state of being unable to see a way out.

Outside of the office, yet still within the working day (the erosion of those distinctions being a symptom by which the present makes and recognizes itself), aimlessness finds compensation in Netflix cop fantasies where rule-breaking is rewarded: wicked actions become the compensatory destination of yet another day's thwarted desires. It's like a cough suppressant: a minor glossing-over, a persistent slight diminishment, a way of cloaking the symptom in a normalcy veneer. Yesterday sucked; tomorrow will be just as bad—at least the gray area between wakefulness and sleep was stuffed with dreams.

The present as a double-edged sword. "And in the austere classical traditions of the Roman Republic the bourgeois gladiators found the ideals and the art forms, the self-deceptions, that they needed to conceal from themselves the bourgeois-limited content of their struggles and to keep their passion on the high plane of great historic tragedy," Marx writes (Marx 1852, p. 5). The impeachment, a reporter explains, "feels like a done deal, like something in the past." As in a sitcom, the pleasure comes in bouquets of knowing what happens next. Is this a second, third, fourth time as farce? The farce reversed into a new kind of tragedy? Realism, in tatters, finds refuge in reaction: from hello kitty to twittercide (on warp drive). The phasers are always set to stun, but always on. Everything happens before it happens, and when it happens, if it happens, cheerleading is mostly what matters.

What is this thing with the radio on all the time? They wanted company—missed their companions, hoped they'd show up. This is a huge risk, writing like this. What is the left thinking out loud? Claudia Rankine's mother told her: "Don't trust white people" (2016). It no longer matters what the world saw, what the cameras recorded. What matters now is "I feared for my life"—what goes on inside a policeman's head: law and order, criminal intent.

And the present can remain in place in the worst way; coasting, drifting—you can't even call it a staycation, glued to the screen. "Beneath the valley of the underdog" (Mudhoney 1998), making sweetness out of filth; finding no faith in sticking to what makes us stuck. Staying up too late again, listening to songs about abjection. Shameful fantasies of heroic inadequacies. Voices, mostly inarticulate between the noises, naming subjects whose entrance into the world felt like an unraveling. The tapestry undone each night.

I remember when subways cost a token and the photocopiers were free.

"Tooled to the same gear," as Uncle George (RIP) may have put it. This is what it feels like, if a car's gear were sentient and even more malleable than flesh. Sometimes it felt like rebellion until in retrospect nothing changed in that direction. It felt like a rehearsal, without the play.

Today on social media someone queer, feminist and enraged referred to "assholes with vaginas." My body responded to the phrase as though I'd looked directly into the sun, blinded by the black spots that I also associate with cancer dots on PET scans, or what traverses the moist membrane in front of the eye when one has just stood up too definitively—a symptom of low or high blood pressure.

I've never experienced high blood pressure, because I've exercised virtually every day for the last forty years. Hospital stay respites don't count, but even there I walk in the halls as long and fast as I can when I can. Most disability is uneven: there are impediments, but something can move, build, thicken, or extend. I learned about blood pressure spots from the socialist screenwriter Preston Sturges. In *The Miracle of Morgan's Creek* (Sturges 1944), an anti-fascist comedy, one of the protagonists has high blood pressure: when Norbert hits an anxiety peak out of fear of masculinity, fathers, cops, and the state, he cries out, "The Spots, The Spots!" Then he falls into a heap or a faint. To him, the slapstick of the present involves self-subtraction, spontaneous disability in the face of power.

That's what "assholes with vaginas" did to my eyes, its hilarious tableau pulling in all directions. Its ambition was to describe liberal and radical women who happily turn their aversions into hates. Hates are joyous: see Rumpelstiltskin. Collective hates make a world. Sara Ahmed notes that haters often call the hate world they make a world of love, because the defense of love justifies hate (Ahmed 2003, pp. 122–144). The historical present follows affect's footprint. Affect circulates, creating a space that can be entered into by the people who believe in its sturdy continuity. The sensed historical present is a promise of a thing we can return to. Concrete matters can follow, the way rocks follow sediment.

Sometimes we're living in the future, because the present is overwhelming. Is there a hole in it? Is the present a hole? The struggle to determine the moment: what is "dated"? (Berlant 2019). Who decides? Political depression: who's there to write to? What does a phrase do? Are our reparative gestures depressive—collecting, exposing, advancing the data story? Testing out the world? (http://feeltankchicago.net).

The present is also a fleshy mess on boulders below the lighthouse. An ugly pastiche. In the shadows below the lighthouse walls, the eyeball doesn't float—it shambles on gluey tentacles, dripping brine, trailing slime. Like all the times you tried to do too much with not enough to pull it off and left an ugly residue. Mermaids with flytrap vaginas; yet another New Prometheus. The monsters are all around us, yet all I see are single white guys carousing unhappily. No relief in duty, rebellion, companionship, solitude, prayer, sex, home-cooked meals. Does the axe come out? You know the answer—but who, if anyone, will make it off the rock alive?

And will they ever have sufficient social density to be affirmed as belonging to some community's world, its present? The movie doesn't say. Lacking warrants, it's too dangerous to name names. The repercussions would have repercussions. The chair tells me, "I cry when I'm angry." They're crying as they say this.

This sensation was brought to them via the auspices of a learning factory that, in the guise of knowing too well, reveals how little it knows. It thinks we're all family. In other words, they loved me for my antagonistic relationship to a labor market I had no business in; when my anger ebbed, their desire did as well. "Warrants," I tell my students, "are the assumptions researchers make, the unspoken rules." A troublesome condition when we're trying to make an object that we can debate, enrich, deplete, or draw. In yet another department meeting, we fail to find a name for what we do. The chair reminds us to remind our students that English is an ideal minor. Skills built there will serve the future claims adjuster well.

In the present we encounter a political scenario that some of us saw coming and others of us voted for, even if we didn't ask for it. TV stars on both sides of the phone call. You didn't get what you bargained for because it was never a bargain. The testimony in the House angered me, when it wasn't stimulating fantasies of a better life.

In the present we need breaks from the present. The pop-up present reminds us that living the way we want to means being able to have confidence that laundry, floor washing, cat scratching, and bathing are breaks like smoking or snacking: visitations of a coast, even a rocky coast that allows us to notice that breathing continues to hold hands with us.

Present-ness, to be present, is an important life lesson, one that I have come upon when seeking a way to and through it. It is the perfect cliché and in no way profound—overly simple in strategies like "breathe" or "be quiet." These always offer an "Ah ha" moment (for me at any rate). I let in and then question these reminders: lessons from the most pop means possible (yoga, Oprah).

I love that the present-ness cat is out of the bag, popular and commodified. The present moment holds in its placebos to offset its offences. Do others also get away from the present by entering the super present tense of a constantly meditative life, where one studies the present and struggles, one sigh at a time, to stay in it? This is a reward for something, not sure what yet, hard work or failed hard work, contentedness or despair?

The first time I meditated I thought I was floating, or was about to. I felt enlightenment in every breath, anxiously. Somewhere to be. Then the wish to sit fell away; then it came back, desperately—if only we could sit together maybe we could recover. Fat chance, pal. My daily dose of frustration. When I write from this idea of a "current moment," I'm describing events and feelings that go back years. Because it is only now that I am sifting the words, hoping to find, or perhaps generate, a thread. My life has been un-thought, many months at a time.

The everyday normativizing of present-ness awareness is historical in its way. It existed before, let's say in less mediated times, when the needs were more direct and obvious, like when I might have needed to go pick an apple in order to eat for the day or help slay the animal that would be my protein. Embarrassingly, I am forced to consider such time travels and generalizations of other historical times regularly with my ten-year-old son. As we hiked in the mountains last week I was queried each 1/3 mile about whether I could, would kill a mountain lion if one threatened us? We discussed how we would do it for the next mile. The conversation enlivened our walk and our bond—inciting clear and unmitigated professions of "I love you" from him and me; our love, the thing that made us willing to. A clever conversationalist, he was keeping me with him—instead of my mind flitting to work, mom, students, aspiration for the future, the past year of outright hurt and, even worse, dull sorrow. He did so by forcing me to locate the urgency of my body and a different mind—one less abstract and variously muddled, one he likes to know exists—in a base act. It's not like this for everyone, but the integration of the two has never been easy going for me; his "what if" questions pull me into a present-ness more simple than I imagine on my own.

For a while I floated on Democratic debates. "An excuse not to work," a colleague says; our reasons for watching are not all that clear, since we know who we'd vote for if they're still in the race (they won't be) and are trying hard not to hate anyone else. After the Las Vegas primary I got excited about Bernie's chances (hating my hope the next week, as the "mess in South Carolina" unfolded). You don't put your money on a number that's not on the wheel.

* * *

Last winter, we watched a video on GRIP (Guiding Rage Into Power) (2019), a Violence Prevention and Emotional Intelligence Life Skills Program at… I forget the name of the prison, but it sounds like "Adderall." It's in California. Medium security, but they still live in the box. They are trying to turn anger and original pain into acceptable feelings, and the program is full of BLEEPs.

Their world is shattering. Each prisoner writes letters to the dead, acknowledges their debt:

> "I want to honor your memory by…"
> "I still feel bad…"
> "I am not my crime…"
> "This is who I taught myself to become."

Letters to the people you killed. This is the deepest kind of repair—there's no expectation of forgiveness, or recognition—but an acknowledgment that the dead are with us.

A present with a loaded past; a present making decisions on a future with peril. Is there a way to harness the madness? The moment of madness in relation to the present?

> One asks, "How do I get fixed?"
> Another says, "I teach anger management."
> A third says, "I deserve to live, to be free."

"I'm a psychiatrist in the rain," sings Lee Scratch Perry. All wet, but still thinking about thinking. It helps a little.

* * *

We're also used to and using being stalled. Fighting for the historical present as a little strip of territory… (Rapper 1942).

> This house is too nasty to be cleaned. We are messy people, and I like it like that.
> Fiction can feel more precarious than life sometimes.

In this parable, Iggy Pop is a big-boned tabby—fourteen or fifteen. A twenty-first century cat. After Adam (human roommate) left for New York and Bone (feline catmate) was killed by a car, Iggy and I moved out of the back room. Gigi moved in. A talkative, altogether public cat. In this scene, I'm up late, Iggy beside me on the couch. Gigi comes down the hall. Iggy falls into a rage. They tangle at the end of the hall, amidst shoes. Gigi's young and strong, Iggy large and determined. Following this encounter, Gigi creeps, tail swishing, only as far as the exact site of her misadventure. There she stops, tail twitching, to yowl from across an unmistakable, imaginary line. She won't cross it even when Iggy's asleep on the couch. Is this what ideology looks like? If so, whose? Mine? Where does it begin?

* * *

From Kurdish Iraq, in the present that we are doing together: if you cannot prove that you are from an unsafe zone, by demonstrating lived knowledge and experience of the place, you cannot move to safety. Hiwa K. tells the story of the person who starts to draw a map of J., a town in the unsafe zone, as if seen from above. Only this aerial view proves knowledge of the town from the ground, but the guy has never set foot there (Hiwa K 2017).

What is that? I said, looking at the images on the screens before me, drifting in and out—a reddish-pink tunnel of circles and little cottony balls. "That's a bit of your stool," said a nurse. She wears bright pink and red; asks what I'm reading, adding, "I'm a reader, too." I tell her, "John Berger's *Hold Everything Dear: Dispatches of Survival and Resistance* (2008)" and "he wrote it after September 11." She said, "the world is terrible, things are really dead." I didn't ask her what she meant, but thought, that's such an un-nurse-like thing to say.

Gravity in the speaking and the ritual of elucidation of the crime and its reverberations. It's a PowerPoint! No, it's a Post-it note! No, it's wokeness! No, it's a tool for struggle! It tells everybody everything they need to know. It's merely a proposition.

And much of what is needed has not yet been invented. We have infrastructure builders. But these days they're patching holes and glitches in the present.

* * *

31 December 2019

My friends Karen and Dwight are driving to Gloucester from Lexington. Karen's demented and needy brother Ward is screaming and crying into the phone. He's on speaker. He called Karen to ask about her claim on a scrawny piece of underbrush in the Florida panhandle, a property leftover from their family's tiny estate.

Ward says he'll vote for anyone but Trump—any Democrat. (He hates Democrats). Ward has been poisoned by politics. His life has been in permanent disarray since he was a child, always falling out from under Karen's wing. Maybe she yelled at him too much. (Don't tell her I said that—she'll probably yell at me).

"Anyway, we couldn't believe he said this. WARD, of all people…" They asked, what happened? And just as he was about to answer, they drove into the Ted Williams tunnel and lost the signal. They both dislike him, having been burned by his explosions over the years, so are ambivalent about calling him back.

31 January 2020

Identity politics can be so good, as an antidote—and so awful too. All backdrop and foreground, no middle.

February 4 2020 (Tuesday morning: 10 hours before The State of the Union speech)

Manifestos are weak at this moment. Certain forms of speech, of theatre, are bound to be upstaged. What if Nancy Pelosi had a paper bag over her head? What if she sat there, holding up her middle finger? What if some endangered species were occupying the Democrats' seats? What if someone let wild animals into the room? Penguins maybe, mulling it all over in their own private code? Or a cloud of locusts, terrorist bugs? Or horseshoe bats, followed by infected pigs, then infected ham and pork and bacon, that they all greedily ate, and expired before the final verdict? We are all so done for...

5 February 2020

She rips up the speech: a meme for the ages. There's nothing spontaneous about these gestures: the soap box, the proclamation, the pinning of screeds on the hallowed door, the rending of garments, the tearing up of documents.

All the air's been sucked out of the room, every room. Even my bathroom. Real estate colonizing our minds. Sprawl, brawling, and cruel.

Amplification is everywhere, as if anyone could hear, as if sound could cut through the noise.

11 February 2020, Report from Shanghai from the BBC's Edward Lawrence:

> It's the end of the Chinese New Year: stay at home...
> Going out on the streets risks infection.
> Wear hazmat clothing, goggles, masks, and gloves.
> Cover everything! Stop circulation.

These are cities without circulatory systems, only roadblocks...
The hotels are all full.

David Quammen says, "You go into a forest and you shake the trees—and viruses fall out." Palm civets, horseshoe bats, amplifying hosts, and spillovers. Can I shed a virus so it's gone for good? Or will it cling, half-life, like a tick? This thing's going to bring the house down. Just-in-time production overturned by the virus. A just-in-time to which we're habituated. The virus as delay, in a time of disorder. And everything is sent from a phone.

Here we go: the pull of fundamentalism, a theory of everything bad... We try to be present for one another, but we fail, over and over. We're either too early, or more often, too late. Some of us lag far behind. And that behind is not a compelling place for others to visit.

I haven't touched my face in weeks. I miss it. Apparently, the President feels the same (Ward 2020, n. p.).

5 March 2020

In Pittsburgh, on the cusp of not being able to go anywhere for a long time. I sensed that it was time to stop all of it. This may be my last flight for months, years maybe. The imperative to seize the present rings more true than ever. I now have regrets. I should have travelled to so many other places while I could, and with Z. Will he see Africa? D's mom most likely died from this thing that is going around but who knows. Here in Pittsburgh for her Shiva. It took place in the living room; the food is in the room adjacent. I hang out in the kitchen. There I find a picture of Z taped to a cabinet. It's faded, just a scrappy computer print-out from a picture of him that I emailed to D. She forwarded it to her mom, who printed it and taped it to her kitchen cabinet. D tells me it has been there for years. I loved that D's mom would see Z each day. I take a photo of *the photo on the cabinet* situation because it will disappear soon. The house will be dismantled—clusters of seating, a card from the Obama family—as they remove G's belongings and put the house on the market. Pittsburgh was not on my list of COVID-induced travel regrets because I was not dying to go there. Nor do I regret going to Pittsburgh on the cusp of the looming crisis. It was for D.

18 March 2020

What do we hold onto when we hold onto each other? On our last day of in-person teaching, I survey the rows of desks with regret. A third of the students haven't shown up; the rest, shrugging, agree to share my mood. Our second week back after spring break, and I had just settled into my new resolve. We've had time to heal from the rebellion a few of them had staged weeks earlier, claiming that the course was too hard. At the time, it had taken most of my flagging fortitude not to scream at them: "You're reading like maybe a third of what I remember reading when I was in a class like this!" Now I saw that I'd miss our cinder block room, with its old-fashioned blackboard and basement windows. I'd miss Anna's straight-backed aspiration and Mike's attempts to attract my attention with naïf comments he thought were louche. The irreplaceable loss would be Vann's irrepressible comments, spoken in a loud whisper each day when I entered the room. She liked to describe me in surprising, slightly painful ways: "Today," she'd say, "you look like a third-rate officer on *Deep Space Voyager*," or "Today you look like a detective who is deep undercover as a college professor." On the last day she says, "you're dressed like a depressed substitute teacher." Such accuracy will be unavailable online.

26 March 2020

Our mayor is blessed with deep tractor-wheel circles under her eyes. She makes quarantine commercials where she's dancing or shooting hoops in the house, but they're funny because rock-hard humorlessness is what we expect. There's even a "Where's Lightfoot?" meme that inserts her rigid body everywhere, like a superhero super-ego. There's nothing light about her foot. She's a matchstick, a deadpan owl. She's the Society after Parties.

The mayor of a large poor city deals with tragedy on the beat. Yesterday the city *only* had 81 shootings, and we're in isolation. Between shootings and COVID the news conference has become a memorial service. She brings the frustrated tones of an exhausted godvoice rather than a joyous performance of how things might be otherwise. It almost has to be this way because the promise that gets someone elected turns quickly into the fantasy of relief called crisis management. People fantasize about returning to normal in the guise of not being rushed or scared. Any pleasures the powerful take seem like a "fuck you" to the suffering. *More* plastic surgery, really? See also De Blasio at the gym. (Mays and Goldstein 2020, n. p.).

A mayor does so much: a mayor could do so much more. But they're all ambitious. They don't do structural change. Their job is repair. It's condemnation and commendation. Structural change is what radicals want. Meanwhile the right thinks people without means should want less. The whole thing is in a mess. People are dying, barely living, living. People's necks are tight from attending.

The mayor is condemned to dirty pragmatics. The President is choosing who to kill. We are not the audience they imagine except when they are scolding.

48°F Cloudy
5830 S Stony Island Ave, Chicago, Illinois, United States

March _ 2020

Hurricane Katrina, toilet paper, precarity, silver linings, unforeseen consequences, herd immunity, a halt to public gatherings, capitalist horizons, Mike Davis's common cold, ingenuity of the private sector, generosity economies, pots and pans at 7 pm, calling someone home, dolphins in the Venice canals, impossibility of grieving, against a politics of wishful thinking...

your shrink FaceTimes you three times by accident, and seems mad, or frazzled, to have been found out. My T.A. was threatened by her employer for wearing a mask—"it will scare the customers."

March _ 2020

With the AIDS epidemic, I knew so many people who were testing positive, getting sick, dying... I was taking care of them, changing Ortez's diaper, touching his terrible sores, we were all so afraid but not of touching, we were all self-educated about that virus and how it was transmitted from person to person.

Late April/early May 2020

Sometimes the future sneaks up behind you. I'm zooming with friends in New York and Chicago. Sharon and Jay have early ultrasounds, which they hold up to the camera: there's a forehead, that's a knee. We wonder what structures of feeling will follow from young life lived in the quar. Are there a million toddlers out there who will suffer the joys of this moment in unforeseen ways? Our confab drifts toward other forms of the unexpected. Alex tells a story about jogging. A biker knocks over a police tape barrier that hasn't stopped anyone from using the lakeshore trail. When Alex pauses to put it back, a black-and-white materializes out of nowhere and the cops berate him via bullhorn. That same day, a thousand miles away, Jay's screamed at for spitting into weeds. Signing off, we agree that a COVID week lasts only six days, but each day's 27 hours long.

19 April 2020

Ballet is back in my life again. The bannister is my makeshift barre. These days I hold on to it with a firmer grip. My legs don't go high but the memory of the movements is still present in my body. I always loved the hardness of it. I love that I never nail it. It is how I learned how to try more than 40 years ago. Trying shows up diaristically for me. My calendar records it. Mostly what I do, it seems, is try.

21 April 2020

> This week I'm navigating my hates and hating myself for having them.
>
> I'm angry these days like a baby in a growth spurt. What the hell is happening?

I've gotten angry at my students' sexism. But why be fed up now, when years of it stain the carpet? Oh right, in the state of the state of emergency there's a pile-up of all the unsaid *what the fuck*s until something leaks or blows.

I'm angry about the stupidity of quarantine-strutting among my friends. The self-inflating love of thinking that the world needs to be taught by your taste. It's not a principled anger: I'm triggered. There's the pain in my heart when I saw the bourgeoisie visibly disrespect my parents. The pain in my gut when my mother turned to little helpers to stay approximately glamorous. The pain in my mouth when I vomited out the feminine chatter that still has my peers of all genders ironing their hair, Botoxing their foreheads, being sentimental, loving that song and lecturing about it, dressing up for zoom and staying very still in meetings to perform themselves as a headshot.

Then I say to myself, get ahold of yourself! (Coots and Gillespie 1938) Why be angry at the spectacle of others trying to fill the bottomless cup of their desire to be held, even by a screen? To welcome themselves to life, if nobody else will? I must be jealous that they're trying.

I'd rather have a good brainstorming session where we keep oh-my-godding and laughing.

Mercy.

40°F Clear
5832 S Stony Island Ave, Chicago, Illinois, United States

24 April 2020

Talking to Tirtza back in January, when we knew the virus was already here: sharing the fullness of dread, preparing ourselves for something we could not recognize, something big and growing, a Cassandra script, but without the words.

Somehow, that alertness made us feel our own small power.

15 May 2020

Each stroll around the neighborhood is a step out of the present. Passing the old apartment, the old friend, the church where my parents married, the site of my father's funeral, the old school, the old this and the old that. There are too many old things. More of them than new things. It is unfair to weigh them against each other. The *now* is freeing but the past is much more apparent.

19 May 2020

When asked, "what are artists doing in this time of crisis?" Hal Foster says, "I have no idea."

When asked, "What's going to happen to the art market?" he says, "I don't care."

20 May 2020

Having lost my job, I'm packing up my office of ten years. The books are easy to put into boxes: a few forgotten friends, a few accomplices chosen for specific courses. I've never gotten over the pride I feel in possessing the least of them. All my life, it occurs to me, I've converted the value of my labor into other people's novels, poems, essays. Although they are in a way extension of me, they don't stir the soul. Turning to file folders of course notes and student papers is another matter. I linger over attendance sheets—these names and faces that trigger no memories. Five years ago, or eight, or nine, I knew them all, had attached a personality and style to each: short-lived bundles of wishes staged for their benefit and my paycheck. Occasionally, a photo stands out, like a suspect in a lineup. Usually, these were the "straight-A" students: those for whom I could imagine books in their future. The rest, I guess, are the innocents; they pass through memory's till toll-free.

21 May 2020

A sentinel event happens in the ordinary.

It's an event you die from that wasn't predicted by the specific way you're vulnerable—cancer, smoking, politically high blood pressure, even. For me, death by car crash, a ricocheted bullet, or the sudden emergence of a tofu allergy would violate the expectation that I'll die from my illness. The sentinel event moots a doctor's prognosis.

We are all living in the present moment of sentinel events.

A sentinel event is what happens. It's surrounded by yellow "CAUTION" tape. It's a sharp shock that disturbs your confidence in your intuitions and predictions.

Last night a friend reported that lab animals are being euthanized lest they die from loneliness during mass quarantine. Then there's the terrible story about the lab dogs who were shocked so frequently that they wouldn't leave their cages when opened. I cried brutally when I heard this on the audiobook. I was running at the time. I've never cried so hard while moving.

I notice that the word "hard" comes up frequently in my writing. I often put it in italics to harden it.

Each morning I wake to the ministry of cruelty. Each morning an anxious putt-putt of sounds passes in the world for thinking. I think about falling back asleep, but fear dying and being lazy. But why is sleep a falling? When you sleep you abandon your attachments. There is no other way. You fall away from hating and cherishing. You fall away from sneering and boredom. You fall away from the drama that makes you feel overalive to a world that's so shitty. And all I have is money, attention. I awake to my obligations, and vitamins.

61°F Cloudy
5830 S Stony Island Ave, Chicago, Illinois, United States

22 May 2020

Mom's cousin's sister dies in Minneapolis. "Of COVID?" I ask. "She was 91," mom says. As a consequence, I'm driving mom's hatchback to a state park north of Rockford, Illinois, where we'll meet a dog walker who's driving down from the Twin Cities. She's been sheltering the dead woman's dog, Rosie. Today, we'll take Rosie back to Chicago; tomorrow, mom will bring her to her cousin's house in Michigan. It feels good to be doing something. We develop elaborate plans for how to disinfect the leash and kennel, dog toys and bags of food.

When we arrive, the dog-walker's pacing back and forth outside her minivan. She waves me over, then demands that I remove my face mask. "Rosie's never seen a face mask before; it's frightening her." My anger scorches me, followed by shame. I'm disgusted by how much I'm disgusted by this presumption of animal equality. Rosie's walker cries as she kisses the dog goodbye. "I've walked her every day for more than six years," she says.

In the background, three park rangers are watching our exchange. Eventually, one dons a mask before coming over to ask us what's going on.

That evening, I take Rosie for a walk. She's eager for exercise, but keeps an eye on me, this stranger in a strange city.

24 May 2020

I've got to do more than feel outrage while watching live lynchings on my phone… or the Amy Cooper video a few days earlier, re-captioning it "Emmet Till, the Remake." I need to do more than denounce her as a racist, despicable pig. In some horrible, festering way, Amy Cooper is all white women's history. We have got to evict her from the house. How do we do that?

His name's "Chauvin," for god's sake.
Racism is always already weaponized.

29 May 2020

Went out early on my bi-weekly trip to the store. The streets were quiet, the market empty of other customers. Got home and turned on the news: a police station burned, reporters arrested, protests across the nation, shots fired. Later, a parade of honking cars winds through the neighborhood. I strain to read signs suspended from their open windows. I can't make them out, but yellow balloons are visible, and streamers on an SUV. Is it a protest? A wedding? A flamboyant funeral? It passes by at a distance, unexplained. I search the internet for neighborhood news, but the most recent results are days old.

29 May 2020

Racism intrudes upon everything in America. Even the present national health crisis, COVID, is infringed upon by racism and the death of George Floyd. It interferes so pervasively and perversely that it leaves people thrashing and banging on things that don't relate to it all, like cars and the glass of store windows. What's the point? Lassoing every object into the story.

30 May 2020

Bring up a tableau of the world. Now erase it, starting with anything Groundhog's Day. Erase until you can't bear one more loss. Look at what remains. It might be nothing or it might be a kernel you make a tight fist around. Your defenses get dizzy from tensing and relaxing when the grip aches.

This season, the 8 year anniversary of my mother's death, the coronavirus crisis, the 3 year anniversary of my surgery, more riotous police. Everything has innumerable backstories. So what?

Not a rhetorical question.

59°F Cloudy
1660 E 56th St, Chicago, Illinois, United States

31 May 2020

Are there anthems for the present? On foreclosure?

> An event may ignite a poem (which may then be labeled a "protest" poem) but not because the poet has "decided" to address that event... a so-called "political" poem comes—if it comes as poetry at all—from fearful and raging, deep and tangled questions within . . .
>
> —Adrienne Rich, "The hermit's scream". (Rich 1983, pp. 71–72)

The present is overwhelming because of what we decide.

References

Ahmed, Sara. 2003. In the Name of Love. *Borderlands* 2, 3. http://www.borderlands.net.au/vol2no3_2003/ahmed_love.htm. Accessed 27 May 2020.

Badu, Erykah. 1997. On & On. *Baduizm*. Santa Monica, CA: Kedar Records.

Badiou, Alain. 2007. The Event in Deleuze. *Parrhesia* 2. Trans. Jon Roffe, 37–44.

Berger, John. 2008. *Hold Everything Dear: Dispatches of Survival and Resistance*. New York: Vintage.

Berlant, Lauren. 2019. Untitled, Untitled. *Supervalent Thought (Research Blog of Lauren Berlant)*. Accessed 30 May 2020. https://supervalentthought.files.wordpress.com/2019/12/jose-cruising-utopia-conference-final-dec-19.pdf.

Coots, J. Fred (music) and Haven Gillespie (lyrics). 1938. You Go to My Head.

Feel Tank Chicago. Website. http://feeltankchicago.net. Accessed 30 May 2020.

Foster, Hal. 2020. What Comes After Farce? Hal Foster & Tim Griffin in conversation. *The Kitchen Broadcast*, May 19.

Hiwa K. 1975/2017. Anecdotes. Accessed 31 May 2020. http://hiwak.net/anecdotes/a-view-from-above/.

Marx, Karl. 1852. *The Eighteenth Brumaire of Louis Bonaparte*. Trans. Saul K. Padover. *Die Revolution*. Marx/Engels Internet Archive. Accessed 28 May 2020. https://www.marxists.org/archive/marx/works/1852/18th-brumaire/.

Mays, Jeffrey C., and Joseph Goldstein. 2020. Mayor Resisted Drastic Steps on Virus. Then Came a Backlash From His Aides. In *The New York Times*, March 16. Accessed on 31 May 2020. https://www.nytimes.com/2020/03/16/nyregion/coronavirus-bill-de-blasio.html.

Mudhoney. 1998. Beneath the Valley of the Underdog. *Tomorrow Hit Today*. New York: Reprise Records.

Preventing Prison Recidivism by Unlearning Toxic Masculinity (GRIP). 2019. *Huffpost*, July 30. Accessed 30 May 2020. https://www.youtube.com/watch?v=GGklV6RD4uE.

Quammen, David. 2020. New Coronavirus Won't Be The Last Outbreak To Move From Animal To Human. *Fresh Air*, February 5. WAMU/National Public Radio.

Rankine, Claudia. 2016, September 27. *President's Inaugural Distinguished Lecture*. Art Institute of Chicago.

Rapper, Irving, Dir. 1942. *Now, Voyager*. New York: Warner Brothers.

Rich, Adrienne. 1983. The hermit's scream. *What is Found There: Notebooks on Poetry and Politics*. New York: W.W. Norton.

Sturges, Preston, Dir. 1944. *The Miracle of Morgan's Creek*. New York: Paramount.

Van Peebles, Melvin, dir. 1971. *Sweet Sweetback's Baadasssss Song*. Yeah, inc.

Ward, Myah. 2020. "I miss it": Trump Jokes about the Struggle of not Touching his Face. *Politico*, March 4.

Correction to: Re/Imagining Depression

Julie Hollenbach and Robin Alex McDonald

Correction to:
J. Hollenbach and R. A. McDonald (eds.), *Re/Imagining Depression*, https://doi.org/10.1007/978-3-030-80554-8

The original version of the book was inadvertently published without the following corrections:

- The author's name of Chapter 11 has been corrected as "francesca ekwuyasi" name to be un-capitalized in the table of contents, contributors list, and within her chapter (pp. 133–138).
- New images have been included in Chapter 2, Figures 1 & 2 (Alphabet of Feeling Bad & Ann Cvetkovich on bed): Pg. 13, immediately following the sentence that reads, "When Karin Michalski invited me to join her for a one-day film shoot in Berlin in April 2012 with the aim of turning a list of feeling words into a lecture-performance for an installation video called The Alphabet of Feeling

The original versions of these chapters can be found at
https://doi.org/10.1007/978-3-030-80554-8_2
https://doi.org/10.1007/978-3-030-80554-8_8
https://doi.org/10.1007/978-3-030-80554-8_10
https://doi.org/10.1007/978-3-030-80554-8_11

J. Hollenbach and R. A. McDonald (eds.), *Re/Imagining Depression*,
https://doi.org/10.1007/978-3-030-80554-8_16

Bad, I had no idea that the project would have such an extensive life across exhibitions, lectures, print publications, and even an audio recording." (Figs.1 and 2).

- New images have been included in Chapter 8, Figure 3 (Ken Lum's Mirror Maze): Pg. 104, immediately following the sentence that reads, "Despite the title of his well-known Mirror Maze with 12 Signs of Depression (2002), I never associated Ken's art with depression, except to the extent that ongoing social inequities based on money, class, race, ethnicity, marginalization or perceived irrelevance produced in him a sense of existential depression." (Fig. 3).
- New images have been included in Chapter 10, Figures 4 & 5 (Vivek Shraya's Trauma Clown): Pg. 120, immediately following the sentence that reads, "This critique of the sanitized, mass-media representation of depression and trauma is echoed in Shraya's recent photography project Trauma Clown (2019), in which she, in costumery reminiscent of a commedia dell'arte harlequin, performs an overdramatized display of misery as she is showered with roses on a theatre stage." (Figs. 4 and 5).

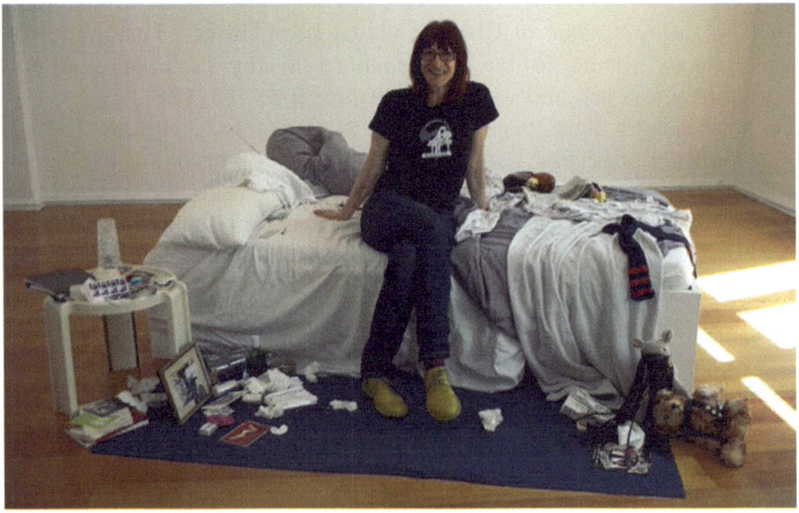

Fig. 1 *The Alphabet of Feeling Bad*, Germany 2012, HD, 12 min. Performance & text: Ann Cvetkovich, Dir.: Karin Michalski, Still: Robert Mleczko. Courtesy of and copyright Ann Cvetkovich and Karin Michalski

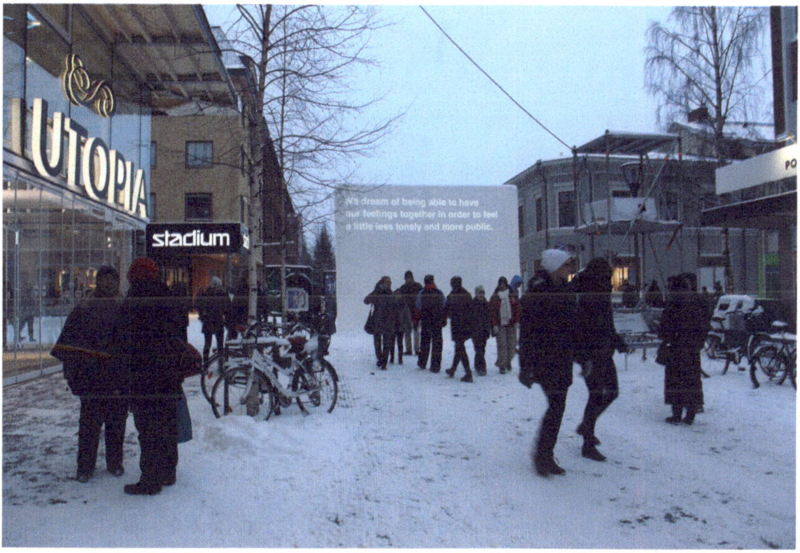

Fig. 2 *The Alphabet of Feeling Bad*/graphic video projection, Germany/Sweden 2014, HD, 14 min. Text: Ann Cvetkovich, Dir.: Karin Michalski, Still/creative producer: Anna Linder. Courtesy of and copyright Ann Cvetkovich and Karin Michalski

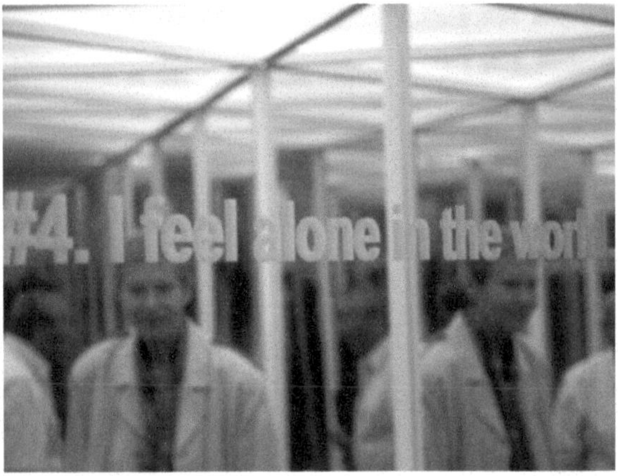

Fig. 3 Ken Lum, Mirror Maze with 12 Signs of Depression, 2002, Documenta 11, Kassel, Germany. Three steel containers with plywood, frost-touched 1 × 2 m mirrors, Plexiglas, ceiling panels with fluorescent light bulbs and plasticized paper, approximately 10 × 10 m. Photograph by Richard Kasiewicz. Courtesy of and copyright Ken Lum

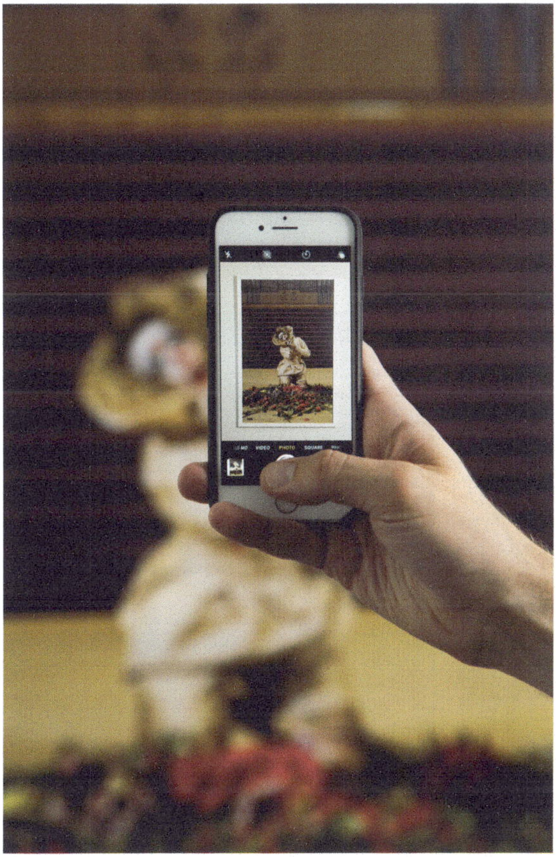

Fig. 4 *Gallery Clown (Trauma Clown)*, 2019. Creative direction by Vivek Shraya. Photograph by Zachary Ayotte. Courtesy of and copyright Vivek Shraya

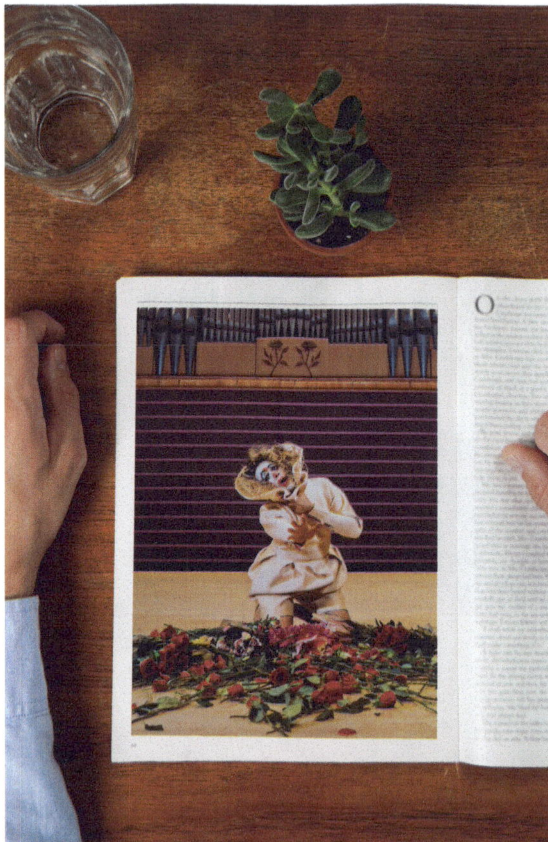

Fig. 5 *Media Clown (Trauma Clown)*, 2019. Creative direction by Vivek Shraya. Photograph by Zachary Ayotte. Courtesy of and copyright Vivek Shraya

The correction chapters has been updated with the changes.

Index

J. Hollenbach and R. A. McDonald (eds.), *Re/Imagining Depression*, https://doi.org/10.1007/978-3-030-80554-8

The manufacturer's authorised representative in the EU is Springer Nature Customer Service Centre GmbH, Europaplatz 3, 69115 Heidelberg, Germany. If you have any concerns regarding our products, please contact ProductSafety@springernature.com

Printed and bound by CPI Group (UK) Ltd, Croydon, CR0 4YY

30/09/2026

02225443-0004